RAPID WEIGHT LOSS FOR WOMEN

DISCOVER THE SECRET FOR A NATURAL WEIGHT LOSS SOLUTION AND AMAZING LOOK WITH MEDITATION, AFFIRMATIONS AND HYPNOSIS WHILE YOU SLEEP.

ANNA PATEL

Text Copyright © [Anna Patel]

Legal & Disclaimer

The information contained in this book and its contents is not designed to replace or take the place of any form of medical or professional advice; and is not meant to replace the need for independent medical, financial, legal or other professional advice or services, as may be required. The content and information in this book has been provided for educational and entertainment purposes only.

The content and information contained in this book has been compiled from sources deemed reliable, and it is accurate to the best of the Author's knowledge, information and belief. However, the Author cannot guarantee its accuracy and validity and cannot be held liable for any errors and/or omissions. Further, changes are periodically made to this book as and when needed. Where appropriate and/or necessary, you must consult a professional (including but not limited to your doctor, attorney, financial advisor or such other professional advisor) before using any of the suggested remedies, techniques, or information in this book.

Upon using the contents and information contained in this book, you agree to hold harmless the Author from and against any damages, costs, and expenses, including any legal fees potentially resulting from the application of any of the information provided by this book. This disclaimer applies to any loss, damages or injury caused by the use and application, whether directly or indirectly, of any advice or information presented, whether for breach of contract, tort, negligence, personal injury, criminal intent, or under any other cause of action.

You agree to accept all risks of using the information presented inside this book. You agree that by continuing to read this book, where appropriate and/or necessary, you shall consult a professional (including but not limited to your doctor, attorney, or financial advisor or such other advisor as needed) before using any of the suggested remedies, techniques, or information in this book.

Table of Contents

Introduction

The desire to lose weight is very common among American women, but it isn't the only thing they want for their bodies. Luckily, intermittent has been proven by research to spur weight loss in American women that were studied, but its health benefits go far beyond weight loss. If you want to feel more energetic, lower your risk of heart disease, and reduce inflammation, intermittent fasting is one lifestyle change that will accomplish all these.

In the four years between 2013 and 2016, half of American citizens said that they wanted to lose weight. This means you are far from the only person in your position. It isn't surprising that more women that were surveyed said they wanted to drop some pounds. While around 60% of women said they had put effort into losing weight, only about 40% of men said the same. Age plays into it too. Just 40% of adults say that they want to lose weight, while 60% of adults under this age say they do. These results from gender and age go across all other demographics: race, income, education, and so on. It has also been found that the more someone weighs, the more likely it is that they say they want to lose weight.

People who want to lose weight employ all sorts of techniques to achieve this end. The most commonly seen techniques are dieting and exercise. As we will see in the book, these two techniques are essential to having success in your health and body. Nowhere in this book will I say that you should not be doing these things.

However, there is a mountain of evidence that the best way to make progress in weight loss. We will continue to cite scientific research backing up this claim. If you need more, you can read through the appendix of studies at the back of the book. The beauty of this technique is that it requires so little change in your day-to-day life when compared to others.

American women have a lot to think about besides losing weight, so a technique that interferes with your life as little as possible is the most practical approach to take. A practical approach like intermittent fasting also makes it more likely that you will continue to follow it through instead of quitting shortly after starting the way that many women do with diet and exercise. If you make exercise your main technique for losing weight, you have to establish a new routine of going to the gym with relative frequency. Of course, all of us could find time in our schedules to do that, but the issue is that changing our schedules so drastically makes us far less likely to keep on track with it. If diet is your main technique, you run into the same obstacle. Your excitement over dieting fades rather quickly once you realize all the planning and calorie counting it demands.

Chapter 1 Lose Weight Quickly and Easily

Forgiving Yourself for Your Dietary Mistakes

Forgiveness is an underrated and extremely important element of weight loss. Often times, people who are in the position of wanting or needing to lose weight fail to acknowledge the fact that they have been feeling incredibly frustrated with themselves. Anger, frustration, disappointment, and sadness directed at yourself when you are on this journey are all incredibly normal feelings to have.

They can also be painful and overwhelming if you do not take the time to acknowledge them, forgive yourself, and heal them as you experience them.

You may find yourself feeling angry, frustrated, disappointed, or sad that you let yourself gain so much weight. You may fail to acknowledge the fact that it was not intentional, or that it had causes that were beyond your control, especially if your weight gain was related to medical conditions or a lack of education around healthy eating.

Regardless of what lead to you gaining weight, you may feel contempt for yourself for "allowing" it to happen, and that may make it difficult for you to truly commit to losing weight.

When you sit in anger and frustration with yourself, it can be difficult to accept yourself as you are now and work toward improving your wellbeing through weight loss. Forgiving yourself for not knowing better or for not doing better, or even forgiving yourself for blaming yourself for something that was beyond your control, is important.

The more you can forgive yourself, the more likely you are to acknowledge that your weight is something you want to work on. Through that, you will be able to work on weight loss from a peaceful frame of mind.

Studies have shown that those who accept themselves as they are and forgive their mistakes are more likely to lose the excess weight and keep it off than those who refuse to forgive themselves. Refusing to forgive yourself can create a massive amount of stress inside of you that makes it difficult for you to stay focused on exercising, eating healthy, and improving your wellness. Many people find that this difficulty in forgiving themselves worsens their self-esteem and self-confidence, which keeps them in the unhealthy cycle of behaviors and patterns that lead to their weight gain in the first place. If you want to overcome these cycles, you need to be willing to forgive yourself for your past choices, mistakes, and experiences that may or may not have been beyond your control.

Another area where you need to master forgiveness is in the process of change. As you move away from old habits and behaviors and into a new way of looking after your body, you are all but guaranteed to make mistakes.

You are going to have days or even weeks where you fall back into old patterns.

Some people even fall back into old patterns and stay trapped in them for years. This happens because they are unwilling to forgive themselves for making a mistake, and so they fall back into the cycle of contempt and low self-esteem and self-worth.

When you can forgive yourself and believe that your commitment to bettering yourself and your life means something, you begin to build your self-esteem. Through that, things like portion control begin to become easier, and you find yourself naturally gravitating toward taking better care of yourself.

Meditation for Portion Control

The following is a simple 5-10-minute meditation that you can do before you sit down to eat a meal.

Using it is going to help you intentionally engage in portion control so that you can refrain from overeating.

Adding this meditation into the mixture will ensure that you are approaching your improved portion control from a deep subconscious level, allowing you to experience even more success in committing to moderation and healing your body through weight loss.

When you do this meditation, you should be actively sitting up with a straight spine. Laying down may lead to you feeling too tired or creating excess calmness in your day, which may lead to you struggling to maintain energy throughout the day.

The Meditation

I want you to begin by intentionally taking one nice deep breath into your belly, pressing your belly button and chest forward with your breath. Then, when you breathe out, let your belly button and chest drawback toward your spine. Feel the movement of your body as it naturally flows with each breath.

Do not try to control the rate at which you breathe or the speed at which you breathe, but instead focus on how your body naturally breathes in and out for you. Feel your body intuitively drawing in and circulating oxygen throughout your body, and exhaling carbon dioxide from your body just as easily.

Notice how calm your body feels with each breath. Feel how breathing is so natural, so simple, so basic, and yet continues to be one of the strongest stress relievers we have. Meditate here with your breath for a few moments as you sink deeply into this feeling of trusting your body and your intuition to take care of you through each breath.

Now, I want you to draw your awareness even deeper, into your stomach. Pause for a moment and notice any hunger that may be arising within your body.

Take into account what this hunger feels like, and what cues your body is giving you that indicates that it is time to eat. Feel yourself acknowledging and becoming aware of your own needs and trusting that your intuition is giving you the right information about your body.

As you start listening to your intuition about your hunger, ask yourself: "How hungry am I?" pay attention to the answer that rises. Are you hungry for a snack or a full meal? Be mindful of how much food your body genuinely wants and how much it needs.

Now, ask yourself, "what am I truly hungry for?" and pay close attention. Trust that whatever answer comes in is correct and be willing to work together with your body to find the best source of nutrition for you and your wellbeing.

Trust that once you are done this meditation, you can opt for something healthier and more nutritious that will help your body meet its needs.

Affirmation to Cut Calories

Affirmations are a wonderful tool to use alongside hypnosis to help you rewire your brain and improve your weight loss abilities. Affirmations are essentially a tool that you use to remind you of your chosen "rewiring" and to encourage your brain to opt for your newer, healthier mindset over your old unhealthy one. Using affirmations is an important part of anchoring your hypnosis efforts into your daily life, so it is important that you use them on a routine basis.

When using affirmations, it is important that you use ones that are relevant and that are going to actually support you in anchoring your chosen reality into your present reality.

What Are Affirmations, and How Do They Work?

Anytime you repeat something to yourself out loud, or in your thoughts, you are affirming something to yourself. We use affirmations on a consistent basis, whether we consciously realize it or not. For example, if you are on your weight loss journey and you repeat "I am never going to lose the weight" to yourself on a regular basis, you are affirming to yourself that you are never going to succeed with weight loss. Likewise, if you are consistently saying, "I will always be fat" or "I am never going to reach my goals" you are affirming those things to yourself, too.

When we use affirmations unintentionally, we often find ourselves using affirmations that can be hurtful and harmful to our psyche and our reality.

You might find yourself locking into becoming a mental bully toward yourself as you consistently repeat things to yourself that are unkind and even downright mean. As you do this, you affirm a lower sense of self-confidence, a lack of motivation, and a commitment to a body shape and wellness journey that you do not actually want to maintain.

Affirmations, whether positive or negative, conscious, or unconscious, are always creating or reinforcing the function of your brain and mindset.

Each time you repeat something to yourself, your subconscious mind hears it and strives to make it a part of your reality. This is because your subconscious mind is responsible for creating your reality and your sense of identity.

It creates both around your affirmations since these are what you perceive as being your absolute truth; therefore, they create a "concrete" foundation for your reality and identity to rest on.

If you want to change these two aspects of yourself and your experience, you are going to need to change what you are routinely repeating to yourself so that you are no longer creating a reality and identity rooted in negativity.

In order to change your subconscious experience, you need to consciously choose positive affirmations and repeat them on a constant basis to help you achieve the reality and identity that you truly want.

What Should I Do with My Affirmations?

After you have chosen what affirmations you want to use, and which ones are going to feel best for you, you need to know what to do with them! The simplest way to use your affirmations is to pick 1-2 affirmations and repeat them to yourself on a regular basis. You can repeat them anytime you feel the need to re-affirm something to yourself, or you can repeat them continually even if they do not seem entirely relevant in the moment.

The key is to make sure that you are always repeating them to yourself so that you are more likely to have success in rewiring your brain and achieving the new, healthier, and more effective beliefs that you need to improve the quality of your life.

How Are Affirmations Going to Help Me Lose Weight?

Affirmations are going to help you lose weight in a few different ways. First and foremost, and probably most obvious, is the fact that affirmations are going to help you get in the mindset of weight loss.

To put it simply: you cannot sit around believing nothing is going to work and expect things to work for you. You need to be able to cultivate a motivated mindset that allows you to create success. If you are unable to believe that it will come true: trust that it will not come true.

As your mindset improves, your subconscious mind is actually going to start changing other things within your body, too.

For example, rather than creating desires and cravings for things that are not healthy for you, your body will begin to create desires and cravings for things that are healthy for you. It will also stop creating inner conflict around making the right choices and taking care of yourself. In fact, you may even find yourself actually falling in love with your new diet and your new exercise routine.

You will also likely find yourself naturally leaning toward behaviors and habits that are healthier for you without having to try so hard to create those habits. In many cases, you might create habits that are healthy for you without even realizing that you are creating those habits.

Rather than having to consciously become aware of the need for habits, and then putting in the work to create them, your body and mind will naturally begin to recognize the need for better habits and will create those habits naturally as well.

You can use these affirmations as they are, or you can adjust them to match what you need for your own belief system. If you do rewrite them, make sure that you are creating ones that directly reflect what you need to hear so that you can change your beliefs to ones that are more supportive and less limiting.

Affirmations for Self-Control

Self-control is an important discipline to have, and not having it can lead to behaviors that are known for making weight loss more challenging. If you are struggling with self-control, the following affirmations will help you change any beliefs you have around self-control so that you can start approaching food, exercise, weight loss, and wellness in general with healthier beliefs.

1.I have self-control.

2.My willpower is my superpower.

3.I am in complete control of myself in this experience.

4.I make my own choices.

5.I have the power to decide.

6.I am dedicated to achieving my goals.

7.I will make the best choice for me.

8.I succeed because I have self-control.

9.I am capable of working through hardships.

10.I am dedicated to overcoming challenges.

Affirmations for Exercise

Exercise is necessary for healthy weight loss, but it can be challenging to commit to. Many people struggle with motivating themselves to exercise, or to exercise enough, to take proper care of their body. If you are struggling with exercising, these affirmations will help motivate you to work out or motivate you to finish your workout on a high note.

1.I am so excited to exercise.

2.I love moving my body.

3.I am focused and ready to exercise.

4.I am showing up at 100%.

5.Today, I will have an excellent workout.

6.I have the courage to see this workout through.

7.My body is becoming stronger every day.

8.I love exercising.

9.Exercising is fun and exciting.

10. I love becoming the best version of myself.

Affirmations for Healthier Habits

Your habits can play a big role in your wellness. From how you eat to how you sleep and how you otherwise take care of yourself, habits are important. As you work toward losing weight and creating a healthier lifestyle, positive affirmations can help you. With the following positive affirmations, you can make committing to your healthier habits much easier.

1.It is easy for me to have healthier habits.

2.I have an easy time eating healthy food.

3.I eat on a regular basis.

4.I choose to eat healthy foods.

5.I move my body on a regular basis.

6.I foster healthy habits, so I can enjoy a healthy body.

7.I always choose the healthy option.

8.I take care of my body in the best way possible.

9.I am dedicated to taking care of my body.

10. Healthy habits come naturally to me.

Affirmations for Self-Esteem

When it comes to body image, self-esteem is important. Low self-esteem can be both the cause of an undesirable body image, and the result of one. If you yourself are unhappy with how you look and feel, it could be because you lack the self-esteem to make a change, or you may feel that way because of how your health is in the present time. Either way, boosting your self-esteem now can help keep you committed to your wellness goals and can improve your ability to foster a body shape and level of health that feels more desirable for you.

1.I deserve a happy, healthy life and body.

2.I am a unique individual.

3.Life is fun and rewarding.

4.I deserve to have a body that helps me explore everything that life has to offer.

5.I choose to be happy and healthy right now. I love my life.

6.I choose to have a healthy experience.

7.I love and accept myself as I am.

8.I am successful now and forevermore.

9.Each day I take a step toward becoming my best self.

10. I deserve to love my body.

Affirmations for Beauty

When we are in the process of changing the way our bodies look, it can be difficult to remember that you are beautiful at all stages of your journey, even the parts you don't like. Having affirmations to help you affirm your beauty to yourself will increase your self-esteem, self-confidence, and self-worth while also helping you generally feel better about yourself.

Plus, the more beautiful you feel, the more likely you are to invest in your physical wellness and appearance, meaning that you will become even more motivated to nourish yourself well and exercise properly so that you can lose weight for good.

1.I am beautiful inside and out.

2.The happier I feel, the more beautiful I become.

3.When I am happy with myself, I am beautiful.

4.My skin is clear, healthy, and glowing.

5.My body is beautiful.

6.I have clean, smooth, and soft skin.

7.I love admiring myself in the mirror.

8.I am a beautiful person.

9.I am grateful for my beautiful body.

10.Each day, my body becomes more beautiful.

As you continue breathing, allow these words to percolate in your mind. Feel them becoming one with who you are, with your identity.

Feel yourself affirming that you are, indeed, a strong, capable, beautiful, worthy, and fit human being that can effortlessly lose the weight that you desire to lose.

Feel yourself lovingly accepting this new, healthier version of yourself. Allow yourself to become one with this new image of you.

Believe the words and affirmations that you have repeated back to yourself and trust that they are true. Commit to believing them.

When you are ready, you can begin to bring your awareness back into the room around you. Allow yourself to open your eyes, return to a natural breathing rhythm, and prepare for the day ahead of you.

As you do, feel yourself believing in every single affirmation you heard today, and trusting that it is completely, absolutely true.

Chapter 2 What is hypnosis for weight loss?

This hypnosis program is for people who want to lose weight, feel confident about their bodies, get toned and be healthy. If you're reading this right now, one thing is for certain and that is that you want to make some serious changes to your body. As a woman, your self-confidence and self-esteem is highly influenced by how you feel about the current state of your body. Make no mistake about it, when you wake up and don't like the appearance staring back at you in the mirror, it sets the whole tone for the rest of the day – negative, for the most part.

You know very well that when you feel great in your own skin, your day just moves along better. You've put your heart into trying to achieve a body that you can feel good about, but alas, not much has come from your efforts. All of this is about to change.

This hypnosis program will help you to:

- Stay committed into trying to achieve a body that you have been searching for all this time.

- Naturally burn up more calories on a day to day basis doing nothing.

- Set up a proper plan that is going to work with your body and help you release fat storage from all the trouble spots on your body.

The book includes:

Hypnosis for naturally losing weight: The hypnosis will help you to change your negative mental views and turn them into positive ones, practice gratitude for weight loss, visualize, accept and appreciate your fabulous healthy body. It will emphasize on how to set and focus on your goals to keep that negativity at bay since losing weight needs consistent reminders and focus on proper mental preparations. Always keep yourself motivated and train yourself to think positive all the time.

Meditation for relaxation: A meditation to reduce muscle tension, lower blood pressure, calm the mind, eliminate stress and achieve mental and physical condition. You can practice it into your everyday life to help you deal with stress, relax and have peace of mind. Deep rest and relaxation achieved through meditation is therefore great for rejuvenating the body to leave you well and mentally serene.

Positive affirmations for weight loss: You will find a sequence of powerful affirmations for weight loss which are intended to magnify your focus on the positive reality you desire and the possibility thereof. They will help you take control of your motivation and release doubt, giving you the power to pave the steps in front of you, as you stride confidently toward your manifesting goals. You are now striding confidently toward manifesting your weight loss goals!

Well, you had better accept it if you want to see optimal results. But as a woman, you need to be on top of your game. To get the most out of the program you need to choose one of the aforementioned hypnosis and focus on it. Once you have finished this program, you should then feel ready and confident to put your best foot forward and see the optimal results that you are looking for.

Dieting plans using to these restrictions can definitely work, but only in the short run. In spite of avoiding regaining those lost pounds, there is a better way to choose.

With the right approach, you get to satisfy your sugar cravings, you get to enjoy some of your favorite foods and you still get to reach your optimal weight.

It should be noted that there are many weight gain triggers other than food. For instance, living in a stressful environment or not getting enough sleep can affect your waistline.

Accordingly, in spite of losing weight and keeping it that way, you need to work on your weight gain triggers just as you need to work on your meal plans.

Moreover, you need to work on changing your weight loss mindset, you need to rewire your thoughts about fitness and healthy living in the in order to stay on the right track in the long run.

Making the decision to lose weight was easy because everyone wants to look good. However, to enjoy success in the long run, you need dedication and commitment to truly follow through on your decision.

This is when things become more difficult as following your decisions over some time can be daunting. This is the main reason why people tend to quit.

For the sake of avoiding this happening to you, in addition to working on slightly changing your dieting pattern, you also need to embrace simple, easy-to-follow, yet effective weight loss tips which will keep you focused and motivated.

Moreover, losing weight is not only about looking good, but way beyond this. Losing weight can benefit you in numerous ways and your dieting choices can definitely make a difference both in the present and in the future.

The best way to go is to follow a dieting plan you can make work in the long run. Once there, with simple weight loss tips you get to stay on the right track, you get to keep your motivation and you get to work on your fitness and weight loss mindset.

These, when combined, lead you towards a healthy lifestyle you have always wanted to embrace, but you have lacked motivation, inspiration or knowledge.

In the direction of starting the journey on the right foot, it is important you understand why you gain or lose weight, what different weight gain factors are and other scientific facts revolving around shedding and gaining pounds.

Why Is It Hard To Lose Weight

You can say goodbye to obsessing over your daily calorie intake, over obsessing over how many carbs you ingested today.

You can say goodbye to extremely restrictive bans on foods as well as on other forced behaviors in pursuance of focusing on getting back into shape in a healthy, natural way by following your body's biology.

You have probably blamed yourself, or your lack of self-discipline in the past. You probably have blamed calories and your dieting formulas which most certainly did not bring anything good your way.

The truth is that there is no one and nothing to blame here. Every step you have taken in the past can teach you something which will help you to succeed in the future.

Another truth is that losing weight can be an extremely difficult thing to do and there are several different reasons behind this.

If you are focused on the weight loss industry, you have probably been told many times before how easy it is to shed those additional pounds.

The industry generally suggests you take this pill, drink that beverage or buy this equipment and simply enjoy your additional pounds melting on their own.

The truth is that the industry generates billions of dollars every year thanks to individuals who spend their money on different weight loss tools and products which can only be effective in the short-run.

Accordingly, many people struggling with weight are still overweight despite hundreds of dollars spent in the industry.

Now, you probably wonder why it is so hard and challenging to lose those additional pounds. It should be noted that there is no magical pill, magical tool or magical equipment that can make the process runs smoothly.

Dieting plans which suggest you completely change your dieting pattern, quit eating your favorite foods and similar restrictions do not work.

There is also scientific evidence as clear as it can get that suggests that cutting your daily calorie intake will not by any means lead to health gains or long-term weight loss.

It would be logical that most dieters have realized they have wrong dieting patterns, but still, individuals set those same weight goals every year.

The truth is that dieting failures are the norm. There is also a massive stigma surrounding heavier people and on many occasions, we can witness the massive blame game which is directed towards dieters who are not able to shed those additional pounds.

On the other hand, looking from a scientific point of view, it is clear that dieting most certainly sets up a truly unfair fight.

Many people are confused to learn that dieting plans suggesting extreme dieting changes, but that this only comes as a result of the statements does not square with their past observations.

There are some thin people who consume junk food and still stay thin without their food choices affecting their weight.

These people most usually think that they stay in shape due to their dieting habits, but the truth is that genetics plays a massive role in helping them stay fit.

These people are praised over their dieting choices as others can only see what they consume, but they cannot examine what is inside their genes.

The Importance Of Genetics

Due to the role of genetics, many individuals struggling with excess pounds will not be as thin as other people even if they embrace the same dieting choices as them and consume them in the exact same quantities.

The bodies of those heavier people can run on fewer calories than thin people require which may sound like a promising thing.

On the other hand, this means that they have more calories left, stored as fat in the body after eating the same food in the same quantities as thinner people.

This means that they need to consume fewer foods than thin people in order to shed pounds. Once they have followed some dieting plan for some time, their overall metabolic state changes which means that they need to consume even fewer calories in pursuance of losing further weight.

It isn't only genetics which makes thin people stay thin, but it is also their mindset revolving around dieting and fitness.

For thin people, as they are non-dieters, it is very easy to ignore those sugary treats and desserts which for heavier people seem like a massive challenge and obstacle on their weight loss journey.

For heavier people, these treats and sugary candies seem as if they are almost jumping around cheerfully making them approach and eat them.

This being said, dieting of any kind causes specific neurological changes which make people more likely to be focused on foods and notice foods everywhere.

Once they notice foods, those neurological changes happening in the brain are what makes it almost impossible to not think about food.

Thin people more often than not forget about those sweet treats on the desk, but dieters tend to keep obsessing over them.

As a matter of fact, dieters seem to crave these foods even more due to those neurological changes.

Moreover, these neurological changes make food taste better due to the fact they cause a greater rush of dopamine or the reward hormone.

This is the exact same hormone releases when drug addicts or substance abusers use their drug. Individuals who are non-dieters do not suffer from these kinds of rushes, so they can peacefully leave a piece of cake untouched.

Dieters also tend to struggle with another issue revolving around neurological changes which affect their hormonal balance.

They face another uphill battle when their leptin hormone or satiety hormone levels go down. Due to this hormonal change, dieters require even more foods to consume in pursuance of feeling full.

This means that they felt hungry following their dieting plans and over some time they feel even hungrier once again due to hormonal changes.

Anti-Obesity Attitudes And Health Issues

It also seems that weight stigma, including those anti-obesity attitudes and behaviors is one of those main culprits of very poor health outcomes in both obese and overweight individuals.

Moreover, these types of attitudes and behaviors toward obese and overweight individuals also significantly contribute to developing different obesity-related health issues.

It is definitely no secret that weight discrimination is prevalent in the USA as well as elsewhere.

It is also not a secret that negative beliefs and negative attitudes about people struggling with weight lead to this massive weight stigma prevalence present across the globe.

This happens due to that common belief that weight discrimination and labeling of people struggling with being obese or overweight will motivate them to lose weight in order to meet those generally-accepted body sizes.

However, instead of motivating them, these people feel extremely pressured to change their attitude and behavior in favor of meeting some ideas which are unhealthy.

The truth is that there are no such ideals you or anyone else needs to follow. You should lose weight only because you want it, because there are numerous health benefits, not because of some fake ideal.

There are numerous studies conducted on the topic which suggest that weight discrimination, does not encourage overweight and obese individuals to improve their health and lose weight.

Instead, thanks to weight stigma, they are at a much-increased risk of developing depression, and increased stress as well as eating disorders and other issues which could have been avoided if there was no weight stigma present in every culture.

These factors, when combined, in most cases lead to even more weight gain, even greater weight stigma as well as serious mental and physical health issues.

How Prevalent Is Weight Discrimination?

It was already mentioned that weight stigma is very prevalent in every part of the globe, but the main question is exactly how prevalent it is.

In a collection of global studies conducted on the topic, the teams working on the project have collected information over the past five years.

They have concluded that more than forty percent of the population around the globe has experienced some kind of weight discrimination whether it was based on an unfair treatment or included some types of weight-based bullying and teasing.

This leads to the conclusion that weight stigma or weight discrimination is one of the most prevalent types of discrimination and women are especially affected.

Among younger adults and teens who experience bullying, teasing or other types of victimization at different places, weight is definitely one of the most common causes.

The same study also concluded that as obesity and overweight rates have risen in the past several decades, the rates of weight-based victimization and discrimination also have risen.

Public Health Campaigns

Even though studies conducted on the topic suggest that society does not consider the influence of biological variables, genes, socioeconomic factors and other variables on body weight, it definitely brings more importance to those less important factors such as the food factor which contributes towards weight gain.

For instance, even when individuals acknowledge that this food factor can contribute towards weight gain, they remain believing that individuals are perfectly able of controlling their food environment however, there is no empirical evidence backing this theory.

Individuals also more often than not believe that people struggling with weight do not have enough willpower to lose weight or that they are simply refusing to conform to usual societal norms.

The result of this type of belief brings even more weight stigma and even more moral judgment towards people struggling with weight.

This trend is definitely driven by the media portrayal of weight control and weight standards which frequently depict people who are overweight in a greatly stigmatizing way.

There are many healthy campaigns addressing the issue designed to prevent obesity from declaring some kind of war on obesity.

Despite their good intentions, their works have a paradoxical effect due to the use of stigmatizing imagery and stigmatizing language.

Messages such as that childhood obesity is a type of child abuse or chubby children may not outlive their parents is extremely stigmatizing and not motivational in any way.

On the other hand, more universal messages such as you have the power to make a change, or you can take control over your health are much more motivational.

Hence, public health campaigns addressing these concerns should focus on understanding people living in a larger body instead of stigmatizing them.

They should focus on helping them the right way by motivation and inspiration, not by teasing and bullying.

Weight discrimination is more prevalent than discrimination based on race and ethnicity and, just like every other type of discrimination, it has to stop.

Otherwise, there will be even more damaging social, health and other issues emerging in the future due to society being unable to truly understand what discrimination of any kind can do to a person.

Heal your relation with food

All too often, we eat well beyond what is needed, and this may lead to unwanted weight gain down the line.

Mindful eating is important because it will help you appreciate food more. Rather than eating large portions just to feel full, you will work on savoring every bite.

This will be helpful for those people who want to fast but need to do something to increase their willpower when they are elongating the periods in between their mealtimes. It will also be very helpful for the individuals who struggle with binge eating.

Portion control alone can be enough for some people to see the physical results of their weight-loss plan. Do your best to incorporate mindful eating practices in your daily life so that you can control how much you are eating.

This meditation is going to be specific for eating an apple. You can practice mindful eating without meditation by sharing meals with others or sitting alone with nothing but a nice view out the window. This meditation will still guide you so that you understand the kinds of thoughts that will be helpful while staying mindful during your meals.

Chapter 3 Strategies and Mind Exercises

When we think of weight management, our minds often go to diet and exercise. What's more important than hitting the gym is exercising our brain. If we make sure that the most important organ in our body is taken care of, we can be certain that other healthy habits will soon follow. You can diet, exercise, and do everything else you need to lose weight, but if you continually distract, deflect, or flat out avoid your problems and root issues, you will never find true happiness. The happier you are and the more aware you can be of your mental health, the better it will be in the end which will also lead to an overall better quality of life.

Keep a Journal

Keeping a journey is a healthy habit for many people no matter what their goals, but it's important for someone that wants to lose weight as well. By writing down your different portion measurements and exercise habits, you can better ensure that you'll have a basis for evaluation. When this is done, you can predict future problems that might keep you from your goals by looking back on the days of recorded mistakes or slipups. You can see what kinds of schedules and structures aren't working so you can create better habits in the end. The more extensive your journaling, the better you'll be able to create your own research study of your weight-loss journey, meaning you can share your progress or use it as a structure for future diets.

Avoid the Scale

The biggest issue with weight-loss strugglers comes when they see the number on the scale. Someone that wants to lose ten pounds might get discouraged if they find they only lost nine. Sometimes, people might even have to gain weight before they end up losing a pound. By avoiding the scale altogether, certain failures and disappointments can be avoided as well.

Find a different way to track your progress. You can have monthly weigh-ins, but it shouldn't be something that should be checked once a day. Our weight fluctuates so much throughout our journey that it isn't worth stressing over on a daily basis. Any checking that happens more than once a day is also likely a bad habit; you're using it to distract yourself from a bigger issue.

The Calorie Myth

When many people diet, they focus too much on calories. They'll see that a certain snack pack only has a hundred calories, which means that it's good for you, right? Wrong. When we focus too much on how many calories are in something, we're failing to look at all the other factors that make up that product. Something with zero calories might include harmful chemicals or hidden substances that are bad for us. Something with a ton of calories might be avoided even though it has a large number of vitamins and necessary fiber.

Calories should still be considered, as the more calories you take in, the more you have to burn through exercise. They still shouldn't be a basis for what foods you decide to eat. If you focus too much on calories, you'll end up losing sight of other important issues. Remember that weight loss isn't about numbers. What's on the scale or on the nutrition package is important in making certain measurements, but they shouldn't be the definitive goals that you're creating on your weight-loss journey.

Talk About It

Keeping things in is never good. In fact, it can feel pretty awful. Those that are overweight might find themselves feeling embarrassed about their weight. Maybe they end up making excuses for themselves when they eat certain foods, verbalizing these reasons to others around them as a form of validation. "Oh, I'll just start my diet tomorrow," you might hear someone say as they sneak a few extra cupcakes from the dessert table. This kind of discussion can be counterintuitive. Instead, try talking about the issues and struggles you have rather than about the way you're going to make up for your problems later. You might find that you end up getting some great advice from a person that's going through a similar struggle.

It's important to be a good listener as well. Sometimes, people aren't looking for answers or advice when they're complaining about their issues. It's nice to just have someone to vent to every once in a while. By creating a discussion, you can more easily tackle the issues that are causing problems in your weight-loss journey.

Avoid telling people about your goal before you get on track, however. Talking about your feelings, emotions, and struggles is always a good thing. Sometimes it just takes saying a thing out loud for it to feel real. However, many people set themselves up for failure by sharing their goals too early. Those that post on social media about how they're going to lose weight are actually less likely to follow through with their goals. Stay silent with the majority in the beginning of your journey, confiding in just those you know you can rely on and trust.

Affirmations

Practicing affirmations is an important mindset strategy in weight loss. An affirmation is a type of positive reinforcement that helps in combating negative thoughts. Instead of telling yourself you're "no good" because you didn't follow through with a small goal, you should give yourself an affirmation such as "I am capable of continuing" to remind yourself of how powerful you really are. Below is a list of positive affirmations you should use in order to combat negative thoughts and improve overall encouragement:

1) I can do this. I am capable of losing weight and I have the ability to reach my goals.

2) I am exercising every day and eating healthy as often as possible. I am actually doing what I should be doing in order to achieve my goals.

3) If I can start my journey, I can finish it.

4) I do not need processed foods to feel happy. I can feel the same joy from cooking a healthy meal.

5) I have exercised before and can do it again. It is hard to start, but I know that once I do, I have what it takes to finish my exercise routine.

6) I am healing myself. I have been through challenging times and deserve to feel happy.

7) I am loved and am full of love.

8) I am losing weight to be healthy.

9) I am beautiful no matter what size. Skipping one day at the gym does not mean that I am not beautiful.

10) I am eating healthy food full of nourishment. I can feel the positive change in my body, and I know that I only have more to look forward to.

Time Management

The most important part of a weight-loss journey is time management. This doesn't mean setting a quick goal and achieving it as fast as possible. It's all about using time properly and understanding how long it takes to actually do something. We set ridiculous goals for ourselves in the hopes that we'll achieve something great, but what ends up happening is, as the end-date approaches, we become overwhelmed and are set up for disappointment. We have to be realistic with our time goals and consider all factors when making different plans.

Practice Patience

Patience is hard to achieve. Anyone that wants to lose weight hopes that they can just jump on the scale after eating a salad and see the number drop by double digits. We have to accept before starting a weight-loss journey that this will never happen. We won't be able to just lose the weight overnight.

Sometimes, patience is hard to have when exercising. Many people find themselves getting bored on treadmills or other machines that require repetitive activity for minutes at a time. Use different exercise methods that you find fun or entertaining, such as a dance class or going on an interesting trail run. If the gym is your only option, use the boring moments on machines as a way to meditate. Clear your head, not thinking of how much weight you want to lose or what else you have to do to get there. Just practice counting or focusing on a quiet place you find peace in, such as a beach or a park. Visualize this in order to find a place of meditation. It'll take practice, but you'll soon find that you can zone out and work hard if you just focus.

There is No Rush

Weight loss takes time; we can't emphasize that enough. Some diets and exercises will help you lose weight quicker than others, but overall, you're going to have to put in a lot of time to lose weight. Remember not to feel too rushed throughout this journey. You have to be strict and consistent to actually see results, but there's no point in forcing yourself into ridiculous time constraints. If you cause yourself anxiety over certain dates, you might feel the need to stress-eat or go through dangerous dieting practices to get there.

Set Small Goals

Instead of looking at a wedding coming up in a couple of months as your goal for losing weight, instead, use that as a small milestone. Many of us get worried looking at the future, thinking of things coming up as the time limits for which we have to lose weight. Maybe it's March and you only have a couple months until swimsuit season. Instead of going on a diet to lose thirty pounds in three months, use the beginning of summer as a small milestone in your journey. Aim, instead, to be healthier and more confident by the time summer comes, rather than giving yourself a ridiculous goal that you don't even know if you can achieve.

Don't Wait for Monday

Many people have an unhealthy perceptive of dieting when looking at certain periods of time. Maybe it's a Tuesday, and so they tell themselves that next Monday is going to be the date to start dieting. In preparation for that date, that same person might make sure to eat all the junk in their house to make sure temptation is removed. But then, by the time Monday comes, something else happens that delays it further.

Even worse, maybe it's Sunday night and you decide that since tomorrow is Monday, you're going to start your diet right now. But then, Tuesday comes, and the diet doesn't start, so you feel discouraged and you count that as just another time that you failed! Don't do this! Instead, set a starting point much further into the future. Find a date two weeks away, whether it's on a Monday, the first of the month, or just a random Wednesday. That way, you can prepare for the official diet-start date. This way, you can practice as the actual date approaches.

For example, your New Year's resolution might be to lose weight. If that's the case, throughout December, you should practice incorporating workout routines a few times a week and experiment with healthy dinners. Then, when January comes around, you have more experience in dieting and are better prepared to actually start your journey than if you had only given yourself a few days to prep.

Something to Tend

Your weight is something to tend. Think of it like a plant. You don't just plant a flower and walk away. The flower will grow, but if you don't go back and make sure to water it, the flower will die. Your journey is a flower. By purchasing this book, you've purchased the seeds. As you read these words, you're reading how to plant the seed and how to make sure that it stays alive. After you've finished the book, it's time to plant the seed. This is done by creating a workout plan and diet.

Once the flower blossoms, you'll have reached your weight-loss goal. Just like the flower, if you abandon your goals and don't tend to your weight-loss journey, you will fall off track and go back into your old lifestyle.

Lifestyle Change

Losing weight isn't just a reduction in numbers. It's a change in the entire way you live your life. There are some people that seem very thin and yet they might be able to eat whatever they want. These people give the illusion that if an overweight person becomes thin, they can then start to eat what they want. That's not how it works, however. Those thin people are just among the handful of individuals that were just born lucky! If you're overweight now, there's a good chance that it's part of your makeup, and weight fluctuations might just be something you have to learn how to manage.

This means you can't just cut out soda for a year, lose fifty pounds, and then start drinking soda again. The weight will come back if you don't manage your habits. That idea can be scary for some people. They might assume that they have to give up soda forever. That doesn't have to be the case. What has to change is just how much soda you can consume. If you drink a Coke a day, you might want to just give the Coke up, hoping you can go back to that behavior after you lose a certain amount of weight.

You have to accept that you can no longer drink a Coke every day if you want to keep up with your weight. Instead, maybe just have soda on weekends, or only when you're going out to eat. Find a way to incorporate the things you desperately love from your past life into your new healthy lifestyle.

Keeping the Weight Off

The part where many people really fall through with their goals is after they actually achieve them! Many people get to their desired weight, see that number, and think they no longer have to keep up with their diet plan. Then, the weight comes back, and the cycle of disappointment has to be lived all over again. Remember that once you reach your first goal, you should set another one. The second might not be as extreme. For example, maybe your first goal is to get down to 180 pounds. Once you do that, you have to come up with something new. That might be getting down to 170 pounds, or it could be something different, such as improving the muscle mass in a certain part of your body. Never stop setting goals. The level of difficulty can fluctuate. But to stay on track and keep the weight off, you have to continually encourage yourself to do better.

Change Things Up

Some people might find that after a year or two of dieting and exercising, they stop losing weight. This can be because their bodies are now used to the healthy behavior. You probably won't ever lose as much weight in a diet as you do at the beginning. Those transformations can be invigorating, but remember that as you continue, it will become a little less drastic.

If you feel you've plateaued in your diet, you should consider changing things up. This might involve trying an entirely new diet, or it could be working out in a different way. Incorporating variety helps to ensure that you'll stick to your goals while also having fun!

Don't Revel in Regret

Once you reach your weight-loss goals, you might find yourself feeling regretful. Maybe you feel remorse over not doing it sooner. You might think to yourself about how if you had started exercising as a teen, it wouldn't be so hard to keep up with the weight now. Don't blame your past self for what they didn't do. Instead, thank them for what they taught you. There is no going back in time. What happened, the decisions we made, and the weight we gained already occurred, and there's no reversing. Instead, we have to look at our past mistakes and use them as lessons.

Remember that you wouldn't be the person you are right now if you hadn't experienced every single thing you did. The more you learn to love yourself, the better you'll be able to forgive the past "you" for all the things they did you wish they hadn't.

It Gets Easier

Always remember that it will get easier. You just have to get into a healthy lifestyle with good habits. The more practice you put into working out, and the more dedicated you are to your diet, the better you'll be able to manage your weight. The first day at the gym is going to be tough. You might be excited to start, but there also might be feelings of fear of judgment and anxiety that you might fail. Don't let anything discourage you from going back. Each and every time you walk through the doors of your gym or decide not to eat the candy in the workroom, remember that next time, it's going to get even easier.

The struggle doesn't end. Your legs will always be sore after an intense workout. You'll still sweat through your T-shirts, and you'll still crave all the sweets that caused the weight gain in the first place. Those difficulties don't just disappear. However, the more dedicated you are and the better focus you have on achieving your goals, the easier it gets each and every time.

Chapter 4 What is Intermittent Fasting?

Fasting has become a hot topic as of late. The buzz around intermittent fasting, in particular, opened a door for many women who wanted to lose weight but were worried about the heavy commitment of a day-long water-only fast. It's hard to say exactly what intermittent fasting is because there are a variety of ways to go about it. When you do an intermittent fast, you are going back and forth in a regular cycle between fasting and eating normally. I will cover all types of IF (the abbreviation for intermittent fasting) in this book, and you can decide which best suits your stage in life and goals.

Many women have seen real change happen in their health, thanks to IF. You could join them by following the various tips contained here. The first task we have to complete is giving you a broad overview of all things intermittent fasting: what the benefits are, what the science says, what different kinds of intermittent fasting exist, and what foods you should eat when you intermittent fast.

We can start with the health benefits. Women who follow a routine of intermittent fasting feel that they have more energy, burn more fat, and lower their chances of getting diabetes or heart disease. Researchers looking into IF find that its practitioners have higher success rates than people who do extended, interrupted fasts and people who use exercise as their chief method to lose weight. They suggest the success of IF is because it can be woven seamlessly into the participants' lives without their having to change multiple aspects of their normal routines.

Intermittent fasting eliminates the perfectionism that sometimes ruins other weight loss techniques. IF doesn't ask that you constantly pay attention to the number of calories you consume. It doesn't punish you harshly for falling out of it for one day.

We will learn more about the science underlying IF later on but suffice to say that you can earn the positive health effects of autophagy without doing extended fasts. The experiments studying people doing IF consistently demonstrate that they see good results from only doing IF, without doing more demanding fasts such as extended water fasting.

This is precisely what IF entails. Nutrition is still important, but regardless of what you eat, you will still see some amount of positive change from IF.

I hope that I have at least made you curious about getting these results from IF in your own life — and to do that, you will need to find a way to implement IF in a way that works for you. It's time to answer the question directly: in the simplest terms, what do I have to do to start intermittent fasting today? What is required of me to start seeing these effects on my health?

Because of the nature of IF, you will, unfortunately, have to start tomorrow, not today — unless it is morning right now. Ask yourself how many hours you think you can fast tomorrow. Let's say it is 6 hours. Most people start their fast after lunch and break it for dinner. Keep in mind that you will have to eat lunch relatively early so that you do not have dinner too late. If you have dinner too late, your system will take hours to start up autophagy while you sleep because you will still be digesting food. You should be able to see now why many women find they are able to succeed in losing weight with IF when they were not successful using other methods. What I described in the last paragraph is all that IF amounts to on your end.

Of course, practice is always harder than theory. I will never tell you that intermittent fasting takes no willpower and resistance on your end. Compared to other potential options, though, IF is extremely straightforward. Still, you might have a long way to go to be ready to live by IF. Maybe you still need to be convinced by the number of studies that we will cover proving the health benefits. Maybe you are scientifically minded and need to learn more about autophagy.

You might get inspired when I tell you all the delicious foods you can eat when you intermittent fast to make autophagy even stronger; you might be ready to start after you read about all the different kinds of IF, and you find the one that is perfect for you.

This one will give you a general idea of all of them so you can keep reading with an informed picture of what you are getting into. You may even choose to check the Table of Contents and read the topic that interest you the most first. It is your choice. Just be sure to read through all of them at some point, so you don't miss any important knowledge.

Intermittent Fasting: Looking at its Effects on Health More Closely

In few words, IF helps you lose weight using short-term and long-term strategies, by depriving your system of calories so you accumulate less fat in the short term and by detoxifying your cells in the long term through autophagy. The short-term strategy is what tends to draw women in, but the long-term strategy is what makes IF great for your body overall.

This is not the same kind of detox that you may be sick of hearing about online. The autophagy triggered by IF is a detox that has always existed in biology and can simply be jumpstarted naturally by fasting. While a detox like "juicing" will claim to clean out your system, supporters of juice diets have no data to back up this assertion. Meanwhile, autophagy has been studied by scientists and nutritionists for decades now. We know that it works to lose weight. We know that it does so without hurting your body the way that other methods do — not only does it not hurt your body, but it has long-term positive consequences like less inflammation and lower cholesterol.

Every organism on the planet goes through autophagy, so you are not even putting your body through anything strange to get these effects on your health. If you had never heard of the word autophagy before, it would still occur in your body. By learning how to trigger autophagy through intermittent fasting, you are simply learning how to optimize it. Autophagy doesn't involve any strange medicines or foods. Whatever you put into your body; you can still trigger autophagy with IF.

Of course, your diet does affect how powerful your autophagy is, but we will talk about that in a moment. For now, I want to tell you more about the short-term effects of IF. The first we will explore is the enhanced health of your skin. The first layer of skin that you have is called the epidermis. You see your epidermis every day because this is the visible part of your skin. There are layers of skin below it, but you don't see those layers unless you suffer an injury.

Both parts of the English word "autophagy" are of Greek origin. "Auto" has the meaning "self" (which you might already know) and "phagy" has the meaning "eat." Put the two together, and you get the fundamental concept of autophagy. Your cells "eat themselves" when they are under acute stress. Unlike you, your cells need energy constantly — even when you are sleeping. They will get it from whatever source they can find. Even when you are not putting food into your body (even when you are fasting), your cells find ways of getting energy. When in this state of stress, their main sources of energy are the following: cell organelles that stopped working, proteins that are no longer being used, and toxins that came from outside your body.

For your first fast, you will notice big changes in your body after only a day. These drastic changes are thanks to autophagy. I guarantee you the first change you will notice is in your skin. It will remind you of when you were younger because of its newfound elasticity and glow. These improvements in your skin are because of autophagy. On an invisible level of your skin pores, your skin cells are cleaning out the toxins described above. On the massive scale of your whole pore, that makes a huge difference. The autophagy results in skin that isn't filled with cellular waste.

The cleaning out of cellular waste isn't the only reason your skin gets better. It's also because you have an increase in the collagen protein in your skin. Collagen is a protein that your skin cells make more of when you are younger. Collagen is the reason the skin of younger people looks the way it is. As you get older, your skin cells make less collagen because they are less effective. This is where autophagy changes everything. Autophagy does two things to make new, young cells: (1) builds them from scratch using the raw materials obtained from eating their own cellular waste or (2) renovates existing cells with new organelles constructed with raw materials obtained from eating their own cellular waste.

Everything should be coming together with intermittent fasting and autophagy now. It all goes like this: you do even a moderate level of fasting that increases your autophagy and then when your skin cells go through autophagy, they make younger cells or make existing cells like younger cells.

The best part is that the improved health of your skin is only the beginning. The main reason everyone who does IF does it is because they want to lose weight. Fasting proves time and time again that it is the best way of doing it. This point has already been driven home, so I will add just one extra point to it: you won't just lose weight, but you will be able to relax about loose skin as well.

The infamous "skin curtain" is the excess skin that people are afraid of getting when they lose weight. It is astonishing how many people say they don't want to lose weight out of fear of loose skin. The good news is that autophagy comes to the rescue on this front. By losing weight through fasting, you cut down on calories and trigger autophagy at the same time. Autophagy's job is to break down poorly performing cells and replace them with new, young cells, or at least replace their organelles with new ones. That's why people who lose weight through fasting are proven to deal with far fewer issues with loose skin. Not only do they have less loose skin to deal with in the beginning, but they are better able to manage what loose skin they do have because of the better health of their skin.

I told you that you would have more energy when you did intermittent fasting, and now it's time to explain the scientific reason why. Autophagy is behind it, as usual. Maybe you have already deduced why by now. The short answer is that the autophagy that IF triggers makes your cells more efficient, and more efficient cells means more energy for you.

As you get older, your cells are less effective than they used to be. They are littered with cellular waste and their cell organs (organelles) are damaged and ineffective in themselves. Autophagy is the remedy to this problem. Autophagy disposes of organelles that aren't performing optimally and disposes of cellular waste and misfolded proteins that are taking up space in your cells without doing anything useful. When all of your cells go through autophagy regularly and take care of these issues, you have more energy because your cells make up all of you, and that makes your system more efficient with energy overall.

Now let's go in more detail on the long-term positive health effects of autophagy triggered through intermittent fasting.

There is research showing that autophagy will fight against tumors, and there is also research showing that it will help them grow — only because cancer cells are cells, too. But although autophagy can work on both sides, the important thing is that autophagy promotes the health of your non-cancerous cells, which will always outnumber your cancerous ones in the early stages. Of course, most people triggering autophagy are doing it to prevent cancer in the early stages and not to stop cancer that is already progressing, so this is all they need. Intermittent fasting has been found to be a powerful tool in combating cancer. While cancer, in general, is still under debate as something that autophagy can prevent altogether, the jury is no longer out for Alzheimer's disease, Parkinson's disease, and Huntington's Disease. We know that these are preventable with autophagy now. Autophagy has been proven to be incredibly effective for matters of the brain.

For long-term problems especially, autophagy is a powerful tool for ensuring the viability and survivability of cells. Scientists did not see autophagy as such a big actor for these diseases until recently. This discovery changes everything scientists thought they knew about the biological process. Excitingly, as I keep telling you, you can trigger autophagy yourself through intermittent fasting.

But cancer is far from the only age-related condition that autophagy can address. Diseases of the mind, heart disease, diseases related to autoimmune failure, and more can be helped with autophagy. While we still aren't sure if autophagy can stop tumors from continuing to grow altogether once they reach a certain size, we know that they can keep the rest of your body around the tumor healthy. This can only be a good thing for fighting cancer, and its why autophagy is useful in preventing all these other diseases too.

In diabetic people, there are clusters of protein built up in their arteries. When they use intermittent fasting to trigger autophagy, scientists can see that these protein clusters are cleared out.

Chapter 5 How does Intermittent Fasting Work.

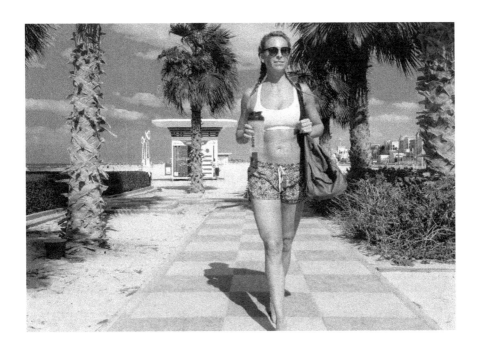

Although our ancestors were aware of the benefits of fasting, they did not have access to the scientific data we have today. In a culture where science is the standard for analysis of what is safe and effective, an intermittent fasting lifestyle would be shorthanded if it was lacking scientific verification of its validity. As fasting diets enter the mainstream, scientific communities are more inclined to research the practice, which, in turn, will allow the general public access to the information and results. A quick internet search will show a handful of studies, and there are surely more to come.

The physical results from an intermittent fasting routine are generally attributed to the calorie restriction that is at the heart of the practice. On the surface, this makes a lot of sense. Eat less food, lose more weight. This may suffice as an explanation for your everyday person, but studies have shown that a more complex equation is at work. Simply eating less and finding your desired results would be miraculous. It is obviously true that other factors that come into play, these factors include your mindset, genetics, stress, and exercise routine. One simple change is not going to completely transform your life. Along with the popular results of weight loss, intermittent fasting has been shown to combat many other unfavorable health risks. This list is quite expansive but let's touch on a few important ones.

Longevity

There have been studies showing that there is a link between fasting and longevity. This has been examined in lab-controlled settings as well as in the greater world. Many indigenous cultures that have a regular fasting routine built into their society have been shown to have some of the oldest living people on earth. Maintaining a healthy weight is the key to a long and successful life and intermittent fasting has been linked to weight loss through a sort of resetting of the circadian rhythms. These rhythms ensure that the body is balanced.

When these rhythms are out of sync, diseases and sickness are more likely to manifest. Studies in mice have shown there is less of a risk for metabolic disease in subjects that had a restricted calorie diet, a phenomenon that translates to humans as well. Another incredible effect of fasting is the regulation of hormone secretion. Hormone regulation is linked to the circadian rhythms but in particular growth hormone secretion is positively affected by intermittent fasting, which in turn may be linked to IF's great influence on long life.

Digestive

It is a long list of beneficial health results that intermittent fasting boasts. The list above barely scratches the surface of the body's natural ability to heal itself with the help of intermittent fasting. Digestive relief is very prominent with newly adopted fasting routines. This is a result of giving your digestive system plenty of rest in between intake windows. Essentially, when we go to sleep, our digestive function stops and rests until we intake calories again. So, if one were to fast in the morning time, they would be giving their digestive functions some extra time to rest and repair itself. Setting a consistent intake window will allow us to build a relationship with our bodies. We become aware of our body's patterns, working with it to ensure regularity. This syncs up with the other bodily functions that we have effectively "reset", resulting in a full mind-body remake, a balance that we can then maintain throughout our lives.

The Brain

We have seen what physically takes place in the body while fasting but what about the more subtle effects? What about what happens in our brain? We should state here that we shouldn't confuse the brain and mind as one and the same. For our intentions in this book, the brain will be referred to as the physical effects that take place in our brain and the mind will refer to our perception and attitude. This being said, we need to look at the brain to fully understand the reactions that intermittent fasting induces. As mentioned above, hormone regulation is a huge benefit of fasting. This regulation takes place in the brain. As the control center of all of our bodily functions, the brain is at the forefront of our health concerns. With intermittent fasting showing such great influence on our brains, we once again find that the beneficial aspects cannot be ignored.

The brain is the epicenter of our entire physical existence wherein our physical and emotional state is dependent on. Seeing how fasting assists in some of the most important bodily functions, we need to reexamine what we have been taught about diet and food. Breaking away from societal standards that suggest an unbalanced and dangerous diet is imperative to achieve the results we desire. We can do this by focusing on our body's natural healing methods. Our body signals to our brain when it is in need. By fasting, we send a signal suggesting that we have no immediate intake of calories. This will trigger the brain to take action, reducing metabolic rates to conserve energy and fat reserves. With no immediate source of energy in the form of recently eaten foods, the body will burn fat reserves. This natural function, combined with a healthy diet and exercise, has shown to be a very safe way to lose weight.

The Heart

At one time in human history, the heart was thought to be the center of all emotional function. Science has proven otherwise, and we know now that the heart's most important function is regulation of our blood flow, distributing nutrients to the entire body. Heart disease has been a common source of illness and death. Unsurprisingly, the reasons for heart disease are combatted by an intermittent fasting routine. Unbalanced blood pressure, high cholesterol, diabetes, and obesity are the main causes of heart disease, and intermittent fasting has been shown to help regulate these symptoms. The "resetting" effect of fasting has assisted the functions of the heart repair and sync up with the rest of the body.

The Liver

Our liver is the filtration system of our body. If the liver is not functioning properly, then, we are left with toxins and other unwanted junk inside of us. The liver produces bile as well, a substance that assists with digestion in the intestines. If our livers are not in check, then many of the benefits of intermittent fasting can be jeopardized. Through the restriction of calories, we allow the liver ample time to do its job. With no toxins to filter, the liver can focus on its own healing capabilities. Also, during calorie restriction, one study found that the liver releases protein that regulates the liver's functions. The regulation and balancing of these natural functions are the keys to much of intermittent fasting's effectiveness.

Other Key Benefits

All the scientific evidence suggests just what many of our ancestors assumed, fasting is quite beneficial, if not mandatory, in the regulation of our body's natural healing functions. This is no small feat for any dietary practice, let alone a free and natural one. Along with the listed benefits above for our major organs, there are even more positive effects from including a fasting routine in our day to day lives. Here are some examples of IF's wonderful results:

- Assists with growth hormone secretion. Similar effects may be obtained through the consumption of supplements like HGH but the effectiveness of these supplements is debatable. Also, wouldn't a free and natural regulation of growth hormones be favored?

- Offers the body assistance with energy production by promoting the creation of mitochondria, the power sources inside of our cells. More energy will help maintain exercise routines and any other activities that require attentiveness and physical movement.

- Calorie restriction leaves the body no choice but to use fat reserves instead of seeking sugars from recent meals to burn. Fat cells are recognized as cleaner energy than carbohydrates and sugars. This will reduce the production of free radicals which have been linked to cancer through the oxidation of cells.

- Reduces inflammation. Inflammation can damage cells and lead to immune diseases and similar other illness. Intermittent fasting can help care for damaged cells when ketones are produced through the burning of fat cells. Ketones help combat inflammation.

- Fasting may also save the body from becoming intolerant to insulin. This may cause insulin to be produced excessively or not produce enough, resulting in diabetic symptoms.

These amazing benefits of IF cannot be ignored. The potential to naturally heal the body and restore organ health is unfounded by any other practice. But with these beneficial effects, many negative misconceptions arise. These misconceptions get propagated online and into the minds of thousands of people, thought to be true, but there is no scientific backing to validate the claims.

Common Misconceptions about Intermittent Fasting

Below are common misconceptions about intermittent fasting:

Fasting allows you to eat unhealthily

Many believe that if you fast sometimes, then you can eat whatever you want and remain healthful. This simply is not the case. Your body needs high-quality sources of nutrients. Sure, you receive some sustenance from a pizza, but these are rarely high-quality nutrients. To be healthy your body needs a variety of foods. Simply fasting then eating fast food in between fasts is not a healthy diet and can actually contradict the benefits of your intermittent fasting.

Fasting is the same as starving

This is a popular talking point for people who advocate against fasting of any type. While fasting can burn stored fat reserves, to be actually starving yourself you would need to use all of your stored sources of energy, and this is hardly even possible to do without getting ill, not to mention that fasting is intentionally restricting calories versus starving which is involuntary. Rest assured that you will not starve yourself if you take the needed measures to develop a safe and healthy intermittent fasting routine.

Fasting can destroy muscle

This is one of the more far-fetched myths in popular culture. When your body has not quick energy to burn, it turns to stored fat cells for fuel, not your muscles. While muscles can become weak and deteriorate in an unhealthy body, this is only in extreme cases where an individual is actually starved or have protein deficiencies. A balanced and mindful intermittent fasting routine is not going to negatively affect your muscles directly.

Fasting works for everyone

Many advocates of intermittent fasting sell it as the holy grail of health. But to realistic, fasting is not for everyone. As we have mentioned, not one lifestyle is going to work for everyone. Many people have illnesses or genetic predispositions that keep them from being able to fast, which is not uncommon throughout the world. Fasting may not work for you so do your research and consult a physician if you are unsure whether or not an intermittent fasting practice is right for you.

Fasting slows your metabolism

While your body will adjust to disrupted meal patterns during intermittent fasting, it doesn't, in any way, "slows" your metabolism. Your metabolism will only be in harm's way if you somehow manage to burn all your fat reserves. This is not a desirable outcome of fasting and would essentially be undereating and starving your body of energy sources. When fasting, we are aiming to burn stored fat cells but using all of them is not something we are trying to do intentionally nor is it something you can successfully accomplish without detrimental health effects.

Knowing that intermittent fasting is backed by scientific grounding, we can rest assured that our dedication to a new dietary perspective is not ill-fated. It is no surprise that generations before us recognized the amazing benefits of fasting without the technology and science we have today. We see that the benefits are substantial but what type of fasting is going to be right for beginners? To reiterate, no one certain way is going to work for everyone, we need to find the method that suits us best as individuals. We will now take a look at the broad variety of intermittent fasting practices.

Intermittent Fasting Techniques

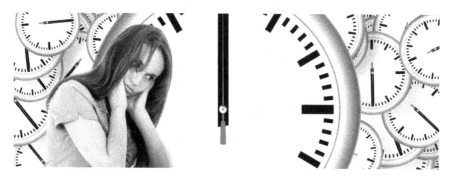

As we continue on our path to becoming our desired self, we must take careful consideration when choosing the intermittent fasting method that will be best for us. We need to again visualize our desired lifestyle and the results it yields. With weight loss in mind, we need to consider how much weight we need to lose and set personal goals for ourselves. Keep this in mind as we analyze the various methods of intermittent fasting, listening to our bodies responding respectively. We should not push ourselves in an unhealthy way. If there is discomfort or other concerning physical changes while fasting, cut back on your routine and seek professional insight from a physician.

This topic will be dedicated to the more popular intermittent fasting methods in the current culture. While there are seemingly endless variations on an intermittent fasting routine, these techniques are a great starting point for beginners. Being aware of our bodies and minds during a fasting practice is the key to learn what works and what doesn't for us as individuals, take time to record notes on your experiences or even make time for thoughtful contemplation on your intermittent fasting practice.

The techniques below are among the most commonly practiced in today's world, keep in mind your goals and limitations while exploring the techniques which are as follows;

- The 5:8 technique

- The 16:8 technique

- The alternating day technique

- The eat- stop-eat technique

- The warrior technique

- The spontaneous technique

We will also evaluate ways to alter and customize your practice. This will allow you to personalize your techniques to align with your individual goals. This is a wonderful aspect of the intermittent fasting lifestyle and you can alter the routine easily, but in the end, the results shine through.

The 5:2 Technique

At a glance:

- 5 days of usual intake typical of your current diet

- 2 days of intake less than 500 calories

This technique is popular among people who do not feel comfortable with zero calorie intake for long periods of time. While to some purists this wouldn't be considered a fast as much as a diet, it is still popular among beginners and people with dietary restrictions and allergies who wish to try an intermittent fasting routine. The technique requires the practitioner to eat their normal diet for five days and then for the remaining two days of the week, there will be no more than 500 calories ingested. The amount of calorie intake on the fast days can be adjusted according to one's comfort, increasing 100 or 200 calories if need be. This technique is a great way to test the waters and see if intermittent fasting may be a suitable option for beginners.

An example of this technique would be for one to predetermine which two days are the fasting days. They can be two consecutive days or randomly distributed days. Once choosing your two fast days, you will go about your business as usual, eating your typical meals. Once a fast day arrives you should have a prepared meal or two in mind that equals your set calorie intake. Many choose to snack throughout the day on raw foods when practicing this technique. Choose foods that are nutrient rich and filling, such as nuts and seeds.

The 16:8 Technique

At a glance:

-    16-hour fast

-    8-hour intake window

-    Eat as much as you like during intake

This technique is well known as the Lean gain's technique and has seen popularity and great results in online communities focused on fasting. This technique requires a sixteen hour fast, allowing for an eight-hour intake window. Sixteen hours may seem like a long time but if you consider that you may be sleeping for eight of those hours it's really not that intimidating.

For example, you could awake, restrict caloric intake for eight hours, open your intake window for eight hours in the afternoon/evening, then sleep for eight hours and you've completed a day of intermittent fasting. During the intake window you would eat your normal sized meal but, being sure to keep track of calorie intake so you can keep a similar amount for the next fast day. This technique is commonplace among people who may already skip breakfast. Unsweetened coffee or tea would be allowed since they contain no calories.

The Eat-Stop-Eat Technique

At a glance:

-   Strict one day fast once per week

-   Usual meals typical to your diet on non-fast days

This technique is found to be popular with intermediate practitioners of intermittent fasting. With the requirement of a strict one day fast, it is often intimidating to beginner, but rest assured it's easier than it sounds. The technique requires meals as usual every day of the week except one day where there is a twenty – four-hour period of zero calorie intake. You may drink water or other non-caloric drinks but aside from that, there is nothing ingested. The time frame you choose to fast doesn't have any other rules except that it is twenty-four hours.

For example, as the week begins, you would decide which day is your fast day. Prepare mentally for the fast day as you go about your typical week. Upon the arrival of the fast day, drink plenty of water and listen to your body, restrict calorie intake for twenty-four hours, perhaps 8:00 a.m. to 8:00 a.m. After the fast day, you would continue with your usual routine until your next chosen fast day.

Chapter 6Common Mistakes While Fasting and How to Avoid Them

One of the most common problems that people face with intermittent fasting is the immense amount of choice and flexibility it offers people. There are so many ways to do it that it leaves the opportunity for "mistakes" wide open. You choose an eating method that works for your life, but sometimes leads to problems. When you decide to try out intermittent fasting, no matter what method you choose or how you aim to do it, a few common mistakes are made often. One of the most common problems is giving up too soon. Others do not regulate their "feasting" meals properly, eating too much or too little when they have the opportunity or not eating "good" foods. Some people fall into the trap of going in too aggressively and trying to push their body to the limit. There are other common mistakes that occur, but no matter what happens, always remember that you can start back at the beginning if you need to!

The most common mistake people make when beginning and sticking to an intermittent fast is giving up early in the process. It is not easy. There will be times when it is uncomfortable. No matter what style of intermittent fasting you choose, it consists of reducing what you eat, breaking your habits, and making different choices. All of this is hard and difficult. You need discipline and commitment. And these traits need to be strong when the hunger hits. Keep in mind that as your body adapts to your new eating style, you will experience "growing" or "adjusting" pains. You may feel irritable and fatigued the first week or two, but once your nobody adjusts, you will notice less and less of this. So, when you are dragging your feet to bed early one night, mumbling to yourself about how ridiculous this is and you should just have that chocolate bar in the pantry, remember that this is going to pass and pass soon. And if you give it two or three weeks and the feelings are still there, then dial back the plan for now. It is possible that the method and structure you have chosen doesn't suit you where you are at right now. Back off a bit, give your body a break and try a new approach. Just don't give up! Keep working towards your goals. You can do this!

The food you consume on your feasting days is another common mistake. Now, there is a caveat here. Many times, when you begin intermittent fasting, you are just focused on completing a fast, not on the food you are eating on a feast day. But if you have seen success for a few weeks, then it's time for you to start examining how you eat during those non-fasting moments. When you start looking into your caloric consumption and the nutritional components for your meals, you may find yourself falling into one of the common "mistake" categories: eating too much, not eating enough, or eating the "wrong" foods. When you break a fast, especially in the beginning, your body may be sending some pretty powerful messages that you need to eat, right now, anything and everything you can get your hands on. You may find yourself consuming your entire days' worth of calories in just one sitting! In the beginning, do not worry too much about this unless it makes you ill and uncomfortable. Instead, celebrate your win of the fast and worry about your food later. When "later" comes, however, you need to take a look at your habits. Ideally, you want to catch your "mistakes" with food earlier, so they do not become something hard to break, but rather a small tweak or adjustment. People looking to lose weight will find it hard to see the big gains they want if they are eating too much when they break their fast. If you are willing to wait to see the pounds slide off, this is good, but it can be very unmotivating for many. Instead, making sure you do not overeat on your feasting days is critical to helping you lose the weight and keep it off.

It is common to find yourself in a situation where your "eyes are bigger than your stomach", meaning that your body feels that it is so hungry it needs much more than it can physically hold. Remember, losing weight is about bringing in fewer calories than you are putting out. To help make sure you get this, try planning and portioning out your meals ahead of time. This way it is a "grab-and-go" type of situation, with the "right" amount of calories for your normal life.

You can manually track what you eat as well. Watching the nutrients and calories of the foods and drinks you are consuming provides powerful information about your progress towards your goals. If you do not want to keep a paper journal of your meals, consider an online resource or app to support you. This way you know exactly how your intake is stacking up against your output. This resource also helps you recognize where you need to cut back on and where you need to beef up for optimal health and weight benefits.

In addition, when you sit down to eat, give yourself time to savor your meal. Try starting the meal off with a glass of water, and then pause between bites and courses, if applicable. It takes time for your body to recognize it is full. If you begin shoveling down the food as soon as you sit down, you deny your brain the time to read the messages from the stomach. Give yourself the time to listen to your body so you can tell the difference between wanting more and needing more.

The other side of the coin are the people that continue their fast when they are supposed to break it. The idea many explain is that they do not want to "undo" what they had done during their non-eating period. People may also think that if they eat too much, the next fast will be harder to accomplish. The problem with this is that your body moves from ketosis to starvation ketosis this way. If you deny your body the nutrients it needs to function properly, eventually, it runs out of fat storage and goes into true "emergency" mode. When you get into this state, your metabolism slows down so much it can almost appear to be stopped. Now, you went from burning fat for fuel to storing it up again. Remember that your body needs a good amount of food—it is called a "feast" day for a reason! Without enough sustenance your body will not function properly, your brain will become cloudy, and you will not have the same "personality" as you did when you had nutrition coming in.

It is normal to feel irritable, weak, tired, and cloudy when you are fasting, but when you reintroduce food, you should see those symptoms dissipate. If they persist, chances are you are not giving your body enough calories. Like overeating, under eaters can benefit from tracking their food and drink intake to identify the areas that they need to ramp up or cut back on. For example, eating a lot of junk food and not enough whole foods can rob your body of the nutrients it needs. A manual food journal or an online resource or application is a great way to make sure you get what you need.

This leads to the third part of food mistakes: choosing to eat the "wrong" foods. When you stop eating food all the time, the food you eat becomes that much more important. This goes beyond just counting your calories. Now, you are diving into the nutrients of food and your dietary needs, and you are starting to find foods within your calorie range but also pack the most nutrients in. A great example is an avocado. It has 500 calories, but the nutrition it provides to the body, such as a good source of "healthy" fat, is a much better choice for your body than a processed bag of pretzels that is also 500 calories. Same calories, much different impact on your body! When you are ready to start diving into your nutrition, this is a great place to examine and refine. Fill your meals and snacks on feasting days with good carbs, lean protein sources, and healthy fats. Choose whole foods over processed ones. And do not forget fiber! This is a great addition that helps with digestion, including bloating and gas. If you can choose mostly healthy foods for your meals and non-fasting days, you help support your body's overall health and weight goals better than ignoring what you put in your mouth. But that being said, enjoying a warm chocolate chip cookie or a salty snack every now and then is not the end of the world!

And, while on the subject of healthy choices, make sure you always have water handy. If you are sick or bored of still water, swap it out for sparkling water or toss some fresh fruit in there to flavor it up. And you also do not need to only drink water while fasting. No, you cannot have a latte or a double chocolate frappuccino with extra drizzle and extra whip with extra everything else. But you can have a good, hot cup of black coffee or herbal tea. You do not want to add anything to it that will introduce calories into your fast, but you can sip on something flavorful, which can often trick your brain into thinking it has gotten it's wanted sustenance. In addition, the mind often mixes up the signal for thirst with the signal for hunger. What you may be feeling is not really hunger, but you are thirsty and need water. The more you drink during a fasting day, the better you will do and the better you will feel. A good idea is to invest in a pretty and functional water bottle that you can take around with you all the time. Keep filling it up when it gets low or empty and make sure you sip on it regularly. If you really need to, set reminders on your phone or alarms for times of the day to keep you drinking often. If you ever experience a fasting day with little water and then compare it to fasting days when you had good hydration, you will notice a dramatic difference in your experience. Hopefully, you will just trust this and not try that out for yourself!

Intermittent fasting is not starvation. These are two different phases of food consumption, although your mind may not always recognize it when you are hungry on your fasting day. The reality, however, is you need food to survive. When you take away food too much, you negatively impact your life, which is the opposite of the intention behind intermittent fasting. Fasting mimics the evolutionary wiring in the brain that dates back to the Paleolithic era; it is a healthy and natural process. Starvation is not. This means your body starts to shut down, including your brain. If you find yourself pushing your fast to be longer, more frequent, and with less and less food, you will probably start to notice continual problems with your everyday functioning. You are also probably entering into disorder "territory". You do not need to overdo it. Find a good place to rest that is sustainable for the long-term and that supports your health goals and healthy weight. Do not fall into this trap of pushing too hard and too far. It is about balance and health, not a competition who can live the longest without eating food. No one wins that competition.

Finally, the last mistake almost all people face, no matter the method of Intermittent fasting chosen, is trying to fit a "square peg in a round hole". What this means is that if you are absolutely miserable and ridiculous while fasting and cannot find a suitable plan that fits your life, do not try to force it into your lifestyle. It is not always the best solution for everyone. Sometimes, it is your plan or the process or adapting to fat burning; sometimes, it is just your body composition. You may have a health issue that does not do well with fasting, like type 1 diabetes, or maybe your lifestyle does not allow or need for caloric restrictions, such as extremely active athletes and physical fitness experts. These people may need a constant supply of energy because their body does not have a lot of stored fat, and they are constantly using their incoming energy. Yes, intermittent fasting reinforces the way most bodies are designed to eat, but not all bodies are the same, and there have been a "few" environmental changes to our world since the Paleolithic era that can also impact your ability to fast.

In some traditions, people are designated into different body types that respond to fasting in different ways. For example, in the Ayurvedic tradition, there are three different types of people. The Kaphic body is more suitable to skipping breakfast but tends to hold on to fat more and can have a sluggish metabolism. On the other hand, a Vata body has a more-flighty meal pattern naturally, making it easy to fast sometimes and disorientating other times. The third body type, Pitta, usually have strong digestion and metabolism, requiring a constant supply of food for energy. This means fasting could throw their natural body functions off balance instead of supporting it. In addition, Pittas tend to be very competitive, turning a standard intermittent fast into a competition. And like mentioned above, this is not always a good thing when dealing with the fuel source for proper body function.

Intermittent fasting should bring balance and health to your life. If you find that you are just miserable every time you "have" to fast, it is okay to ask yourself if the benefits of the fast are greater than the quality of life and happiness you are sacrificing. If you find that the misery is greater than the results, maybe you should rethink your approach to intermittent fasting altogether. There are other diet plans out there that may be better suited for your success.

Recall back to when you shifted your perspective from "have" to do intermittent fasting, despite how "hard" and "difficult" it is, to a fresh view of a new experiment designed to teach you about yourself and your body. When you find yourself struggling with one of these "mistakes" or one of the myriads of other "mistakes" you can encounter with such a broad approach to eating, bring your mindset back to one of curiosity and learning. Give yourself permission to experiment with what works and what does not without stamping a big "F" on your efforts. Even if you decide that intermittent fasting is not for you, you deserve a gold star and a celebration for taking the time to learn more about your body and its needs. That is a huge win and accomplishment you should embrace!

Chapter 7 Enhance Your Motivation

"Of course, motivation is not permanent. But then, neither is bathing; but it is something you should do on a regular basis."
— Zig Ziglar1

Your journey is going to start with your motivation level. Many things are possible, but it feels like almost nothing is when you are lacking motivation. Getting out of bed morning after morning, trying to find the strength to make it through the day can feel as hard as trying to climb a mountain on some days. Motivation can be found in many different things, but it will always come from our minds. What we're passionate about, the things that really matter, those are what motivates us to make it through the day.

The first thing you are going to want to do to motivate you is to change your attitude into a positive one. When we look at the world through a gray lens, we can easily see everything as terrible. When you hate one thing, that hate starts to grow and can spread into other parts of your life. We can't look at life through rose-colored glasses either, because we don't want to make ourselves ignorant to reality. We have to look at the world, at our life, head on, as it is in an objective way. When we can do this, it will be much easier to take on the new things that present themselves to you each and every day.

Give yourself time to prepare to be motivated too, not just time to start the weight loss. First, you have to get in the right mindset. Then, you can prepare for your meal plan and exercise regimen before starting. If you try to force yourself into it, you might sometimes make it even harder to get started.

As humans, we like to be independent. Not everyone is interested in being told what to do and we sometimes seek to be defiant in ways, even against ourselves. Sometimes in our heads, the things we're being told to do won't be our own ideas and can instead simply be the pressures of society, our peers, and our parents. Their voices can still get so deep in our heads that we will mistake them for our own and can easily get frustrated with what we're telling ourselves.

It can seem like an internal battle when you are trying to get motivated. There's the part of you that knows what you have to do, and then there's the voice that's telling you to just not do it. To just sit around and wait for tomorrow. Motivation is all about silencing that voice and building one of encouragement.

Don't allow any regret into your life or into the future. Regret can be such a wasted emotion. At the end of the day, it is not. There is a psychological purpose for regret. It causes us to look back on our mistakes and question our motives for doing certain things. Regret can teach us how to be better in the future. However, too much regret can lead to a lot of time wasted. There are some individuals that will be so regretful over certain decisions that it consumes their entire life. If you want to move forward and be motivated, not just about weight loss but with everything in your life, then you have to learn how to let go of regret. Feeling it in the first place isn't wrong, but don't entertain it anymore. Think of it like someone that you pass at the grocery store, someone that that you want to still is respectful towards even though you aren't very fond of him or her. Instead of talking to them and inviting them out to dinner, simply smile at them and keep walking. This is how we have to learn to process all feelings of regret, and emotions of guilt and shame as well. Simply let it passes, but do not allow it to stay past its welcome.

You are the person that you are right now because of the life that you've lived. It can be so easy to think, "Oh I should have done this," or "if only I had gone with the other option." However, if we hadn't made that one choice, then our lives would be incredibly different than what they are now. Each thing we've experienced, the decisions we've made and the thoughts that we've had, these are all like ingredients that go into what makes us who we are. When you can learn to love yourself and the person that you've become, then it will be easier to build that motivation because you'll let that guilt and regret losing.

Look at what motivates you right now, at this very second. What's the first thing that comes to mind? Maybe it is wanting to make a loved one proud or providing for your child. Perhaps your motivation is getting your bills paid or simply making your next meal. Whatever it is, this can tell you a lot about what drives you in this life. When you can become aware of all the motivating factors in your life, it will be a lot easier to use these images and ideas when you are struggling in certain situations. If nothing comes to mind at all, then it is time to do some soul searching. At the very least, wanting to make ourselves happy should be a motivator. Feeling good and looking better is all I need to motivate me on some days; however, others require a little more work.

Honestly, sometimes food was a motivator for me. I would tell myself that if I could avoid fast food all week and eat healthy Monday-Friday, that Saturday, I could go crazy. I told myself it didn't' matter if I wanted to drive myself through Taco Bell, Wendy's, and KFC all in one week. Whatever I decided for Saturday would be fine, as long as I stayed resilient against my cravings for Monday-Friday. If I was struggling on Wednesday and just wanted to skip the salad I brought to work and walk to the fast food joint across the street, I would remind myself that I could get it on Saturday. When I would diet in the past, I would think that I had to cut all bad food out for the time being. It would drive me crazy! Eventually, I realized that I had to give myself looser restrictions and reminding myself that it wouldn't be too long before I could have fast food again helped to keep me motivated throughout the week, rather than constantly thinking about the food that I wanted.

What would end up happening was that I felt so good about myself for eating healthy all week that I wouldn't want to ruin my streak so I would keep up the diet. I would get to Saturday and think to myself that I had done so well all week, why ruin it now? I might still occasionally go out to dinner with my family on the weekends and get something that isn't great for me, but then this was a reward. I realized that motivation would breed more motivation. The easier it was for me to get started with the things I want and stay focused on my goals, the more this strengthened my willpower. There are always going to be hard days, but I just remind myself that this is part of the process.

Your Dream Outfit

"Weight loss doesn't begin in the gym with a dumbbell; it starts in your head with a decision." — Toni Sorenson3

Some people will put pictures of their celebrity icons on their fridge, or maybe even their mirror, so that they see them when they wake up. You need motivation that will help you picture yourself in your future, not someone else's body and journey. If your main motivation is done through comparing yourself to others, then that's not going to be healthy in the long-run. Instead, it might drive you to eat more because you are feeling bad about yourself, in more of a fragile state where you are going to decrease motivation levels. The thing about celebrity bodies is that if they aren't photo shopped, then they were still achieved through trick lighting and a team of makeup artists, as well as a personal trainer and shopper that gives them all the tools needed to lose weight. Most of us women are doing this on our own, so we have to stay realistic.

If you are 5 feet tall and you put a Victoria's Secret model on your fridge, that's not going to do you any good. We all have different bodies, and even if you were at your healthiest body weight, you might still not look anything near to the person that you are comparing your body to. Some of us are naturally curvier as well, while others might be stick-thin. You might have larger breasts and hips, or a bigger shoulder structure than many thinner models on the runway. We can't expect our bodies to look like theirs if the structure and height aren't the same, so using other people's pictures is never a good idea. It can just make you feel worse about yourself because you might get below your healthy weight and still not look like the other person, so you will still be disliking your body.

Right now, think of what your ultimate dream outfit would be. Whether it is a slim-fitting dress, or a cute crop-top and some butt - lifting high waist jeans, think of an outfit that you want to be able to look totally cute in. This is going to be your biggest motivator when you are getting started. You will be able to actually see yourself in this dress and be able to look at it with your own body, not just what someone else might look like. Be realistic with your sizing as well. Only go down a few sizes, somewhere that you would still feel good about yourself getting into. If you are a size 24 right now and you buy a size 0 dress, that's unrealistic. That could take years to get into, and there's a good chance that your body structure still wouldn't be able to slip into a 0. This is a small size and people that are a size 0 and have a healthy body weight are usually shorter, so be realistic. A size 16 dress would probably be a good place to start if you are currently at a 24. And if you are a size 16 now, then a size 10 would be good. Make sure you are aiming for something in between what your size is now, and what half of that size would be, give or take a number.

Try to not pick a bikini or something that would make you feel uncomfortable. A bikini or swimsuit can be good for some people, but swimwear can be triggering for many women, especially those that have continuously struggled with their weight. Pick something that you would wear now at your comfort level. If you try to push yourself too hard, you could end up making yourself afraid of what might happen and could even self-sabotage.

Hang this outfit somewhere that you will see it every single day. I put it on the back of my bedroom door so that I could see it every day when I woke up and every night before I fell asleep. It would help me to remind myself of all that I wanted to achieve and give me the strength and encouragement in the morning to not give up on the thing that I wanted the most. Make sure that you are giving yourself the proper time to reach this goal as well. If you try to fit into something 10 sizes smaller after 2 months, you are just going to end up disappointing yourself.

Studies on Habit

We all have different habits that we do. Some people have a habit of working out every day, others have a habit of eating a candy bar every night. Whatever it is, there are certain things that we do ritualistically. Sometimes, we don't even realize that what we are doing is a habit. Our brains can become so accustomed to doing the same thing over and over again that we won't always recognize when we've adopted behavior that is consistent and harder to break. Instead, we have to look at others to remind us of our habits and point out the things that we consistently do.

Habit forming actually starts within the neurology of our brains. When you are learning something, you take it in and process it in a certain way. Your brain takes the information and decides if it wants to store it in the long-term or short-term memory. You learn what you can from each experience and then your brain moves onto other things. It does this when learning or doing all new things. After repeatedly taking in that same information, your brain will no longer process it the same. Your brain just won't give it the same amount of energy. It becomes second nature because your brain doesn't think there's anything valuable to get from it. For example, you might have a habit of going for a walk every day. On that first walk, your brain took in that information, and you noticed everything new. The houses along the path, the marks in the sidewalk, the biggest trees, you noticed all this kind of stuff. Then, as you kept going on the same walk, on that same route, your brain stopped looking for something new. It became a habit.

Habits will give us the ability to put our attention on something else4. If we were constantly alert and paying attention to all the details of everything we see and experience, then it can be very overwhelming for our brains. We can even go through sensory overload. We need to take a break sometimes and just do the mindless things, so our consciousness isn't always working so hard. However, if everything becomes a habit, then our brains will also stop evolving and growing.

We have to start recognizing our habits if we ever want them to change. This can be hard, but it just requires you to be mindful throughout the day. before doing anything, ask yourself why you're doing it. Even if it's simply going to the bathroom. As you stand up from the couch to go pee once you get that feeling in your bladder, recognize what you are doing, why you're doing it, and the motivation behind it. When we can practice mindful living in all aspects of our lives, then it becomes easier to do so more naturally. Motivation can build the desire to change your intentions, but it is only up to you to actually change the outcome. You might get the fantasy or exciting idea to lose the weight and go on a diet. However, actually going through with that will require you to recognize and break your worst habits.

Just like you took a little while to form a habit, it is going to take a bit to get it to go away. You won't be able to just stop the habit overnight. Your brain was trained to do this! Have you ever tried to brush your teeth with the opposite hand? It can be challenging! Remember that you aren't just habitual for no reason. You can look deep inside yourself to see what drives you and do your best to break those bad habits.

Research on Motivation

We need motivation to do literally anything. A lot of times, we don't realize the motivation behind certain actions. How many times have you reflected on something you've done and thought, "Why on Earth did I just do that?" Though we feel like we're in charge often, there are a lot of times when it feels like we have almost no control at all. This is because sometimes, our subconscious will think it knows what's best for us better than we would of ourselves. The better we can understand our own motivation on an individual level, the easier it will be to create those feelings of encouragement within ourselves. Those that struggle with weight loss aren't the only ones who are concerned with motivation either. Since it is so relevant in all aspects of life, we have scientific research that allows us insight into what might drive our most basic desires.

We have two different kinds of goals when it comes to motivation, mastery and performance5. On one hand, you might desire to achieve something because you want to master that task.

Your Reason for Motivation

Finding a solid reason to lose weight is something that's going to be very important in your journey. On one hand, you won't want to do it just for other people. This is something that you have to do for yourself. If you want to make your spouse, children, peers, parents, or anyone else proud, that's great! But you have to remember that what will matter most in this journey is making yourself proud.

Competition can be helpful, but at first, you just need to focus on yourself, especially if this has been a long journey for you. If you're too competitive, then you might make yourself feel bad. Competition should be fun and encouraging, like doing a small race with a friend. If you base your life around it and only find worth in beating other people, then that's going to be harmful to your perspective on yourself, making it even more challenging to lose the weight and keep it off.

Chapter 8 Blasting Calories

We have all heard the word "calorie" and its relation to our body weight. Calories are contained in the foods we consume and are often misunderstood about how they affect us. In this topic, we seek to explain what they are, how to count them, and the best methods of blasting them to avoid weight gain.

What are Calories, and how do they affect Your Weight?

A calorie is a key estimating unit. For example, we use meters when communicating separation;' Usain Bolt went 100 meters in simply 9.5 seconds.' There are two units in this expression. One is a meter (a range unit), and the other is "second" (a period unit). Essentially, calories are additional units of physical amount estimation.

Many assume that a calorie is the weight measure (since it is oftentimes connected with an individual's weight). That is not precise, however. A calorie is a vitality unit (estimation). 1 calorie is proportional to the vitality expected to build the temperature by 1 degree Celsius to 1 kilogram of water.

Two particular sorts of calories come in: small calories and huge calories. Huge calories are the word connected to sustenance items.

You've likely observed much stuff on parcels (chocolates, potato chips, and so forth.) with' calorie scores.' Imagine the calorie score an incentive for a thing being' 100 cal.' this infers when you eat it, you will pick up about as much vitality (even though the calorie worth expressed and the amount you advantage from it is never the equivalent).

All that we eat has a particular calorie tally; it is the proportion of the vitality we eat in the substance bonds. B

These are mostly things we eat: starches, proteins, and fats. How about we take a gander at what number of calories 1 gram comprises of these medications: 1. Sugars 4 calories 2. Protein− 3 calories. Fat−nine calories

Are my calories awful?

That is fundamentally equivalent to mentioning, "Is vitality awful for me?" Every single activity the body completes needs vitality. Everything takes vitality to stand, walk, run, sit, and even eat. In case you're doing any of these tasks, it suggests you're utilizing vitality, which mostly infers you're' consuming' calories, explicitly the calories that entered your body when you were eating some nourishment.

To sum things up, for you, NO... calories are not terrible.

Equalization is the way to finding harmony between what number of calories you devour and what number of calories you consume or use. On the off chance that you eat fewer calories and spend more, you will become dainty, while on the opposite side, on the off chance that you gobble up heaps of calories, however, you are a habitually lazy person, you will in the long run become stout at last.

Each movement we do throughout a day will bring about certain calories being spent. Here is a little rundown of the absolute most much of the time performed exercises, just as the number of calories consumed while doing them.

Step by step instructions to Count Calories

You have to expend fewer calories than you consume to get thinner.

This clamor is simple in principle. Be that as it may, it very well may be hard to deal with your nourishment admission in the contemporary sustenance setting. Calorie checking is one approach to address this issue and is much of the time used to get more fit. Hearing that calories don't make a difference is very common, and tallying calories is an exercise in futility. Nonetheless, calories tally with regards to your weight; this is a reality that, in science, analyses called overloading studies has been demonstrated on numerous occasions.

These examinations request that people deliberately indulge and after that, survey the impact on their weight and wellbeing. All overloading investigations have found that people are putting on weight when they devour a bigger number of calories than they consume.

This simple reality infers that calorie checking and limiting your utilization can be proficient in averting weight put on or weight reduction as long as you can stick to it. One examination found that health improvement plans, including calorie including brought about a normal weight reduction of around 7 lbs. (3.3 kg) more than those that didn't.

Primary concern: You put on weight by eating a larger number of calories than you consume. Calorie tallying can help you expend fewer calories and get more fit.

How many calories do you have to eat?

What number of calories you need depends on factors, for example, sex, age, weight, and measure of activity? For example, a 25-year-old male competitor will require a bigger number of calories than a non-practicing 70-year-elderly person. In case you're endeavoring to get in shape, by eating not exactly your body consumes off, you'll have to construct a calorie deficiency. Utilize this adding machine to decide what number of calories you ought to expend every day (opening in crisp tab). This number cruncher depends on the condition of Mifflin-St Jeor, an exact method to evaluate calorie prerequisites.

How to Reduce your Caloric Intake for Weight Loss

Bit sizes have risen, and a solitary dinner may give twofold or triple what the normal individual needs in a sitting at certain cafés. "Segment mutilation" is the term used to depict enormous parts of sustenance as the standard. It might bring about weight put on and weight reduction. In general, people don't evaluate the amount they spend. Tallying calories can help you battle indulging by giving you a more grounded information of the amount you expend.

In any case, you have to record portions of sustenance appropriately for it to work. Here are a couple of well-known strategies for estimating segment sizes: Scales: Weighing your sustenance is the most exact approach to decide the amount you eat. This might be tedious, in any case, and isn't constantly down to earth.

Estimating cups: Standard estimations of amount are, to some degree, quicker and less complex to use than a scale, yet can some of the time be tedious and unbalanced.

Examinations: It's quick and easy to utilize correlations with well-known items, especially in case you're away from home. It's considerably less exact, however.

Contrasted with family unit items, here are some mainstream serving sizes that can help you gauge your serving sizes: 1

serving of rice or pasta (1/2 a cup): a PC mouse or adjusted bunch.

- 1 Meat serving (3 oz): a card deck.

- 1 Fish serving (3 oz): visit book.

- 1 Cheese serving (1.5 oz): a lipstick or thumb size.

- 1 Fresh organic product serving (1/2 cup): a tennis ball.

- 1 Green verdant vegetable serving (1 cup): baseball.

- 1 Vegetable serving (1/2 cup): a mouse PC.

- 1 Olive oil teaspoon: 1 fingertip.

- 2 Peanut margarine tablespoons: a ping pong ball.

Calorie tallying, notwithstanding when gauging and estimating partitions, isn't a careful science.

In any case, your estimations shouldn't be thoroughly spot-on. Simply guarantee that your utilization is recorded as effectively as would be prudent. You ought to be mindful to record high-fat as well as sugar things, for example, pizza, dessert, and oils. Under-recording these meals can make an enormous qualification between your genuine and recorded utilization. You can endeavor to utilize scales toward the begin to give you a superior idea of what a segment resembles to upgrade your evaluations. This should help you to be increasingly exact, even after you quit utilizing them.

More Tips to Assist in Caloric Control

Here are 5 more calorie tallying tips:

• Get prepared: get a calorie tallying application or web device before you start, choose how to evaluate or gauge parcels, and make a feast plan.

• Read nourishment marks: Food names contain numerous accommodating calorie tallying information. Check the recommended segment size on the bundle.

• Remove the allurement: dispose of your home's low-quality nourishment. This will help you select more advantageous bites and make hitting your objectives easier.

• Aim for moderate, steady loss of weight: don't cut too little calories. Even though you will get in shape all the more rapidly, you may feel terrible and be less inclined to adhere to your arrangement.

• Fuel your activity: Diet and exercise are the best health improvement plans. Ensure you devour enough to rehearse your vitality.

Effective Methods for Blasting Calories

To impact calories requires participating in exercises that urge the body to utilize vitality. Aside from checking the calories and guaranteeing you eat the required sum, consuming them is similarly basic for weight reduction. Here, we examine a couple of techniques that can enable you to impact our calories all the more viably.:

1. Indoor cycling: McCall states that around 952 calories for each hour ought to be at 200 watts or higher. On the off chance that the stationary bicycle doesn't demonstrate watts: "This infers you're doing it when your indoor cycling instructor educates you to switch the opposition up!" he proposes.

2. Skiing: around 850 calories for every hour depends on your skiing knowledge. Slow, light exertion won't consume nearly the same number of calories as a lively, fiery exertion is going to consume. To challenge yourself and to consume vitality? Attempt to ski tough.

3. Rowing: Approximately 816 calories for every hour. The benchmark here is 200 watts; McCall claims it ought to be at a "fiery endeavor." Many paddling machines list the showcase watts. Reward: Rowing is additionally a stunning back exercise.

4. Jumping rope: About 802 calories for each hour This ought to be at a moderate pace—around 100 skips for each moment—says McCall. Attempt to begin with this bounce rope interim exercise.

5. Kickboxing: Approximately 700 calories for every hour. Also, in this class are different sorts of hand to hand fighting, for example, Muay Thai. With regards to standard boxing, when you are genuine in the ring (a.k.a. battling another individual), the biggest calorie consumption develops. Be that as it may, many boxing courses additionally incorporate cardio activities, for example, hikers and burpees, so your pulse will in the long run increment more than you would anticipate. What's more, hello, before you can get into the ring, you need to start someplace, isn't that so?

6. Swimming: Approximately 680 calories for each hour Freestyle works, however as McCall says, you should go for a vivacious 75 yards for each moment. For an easygoing swimmer, this is somewhat forceful. (Butterfly stroke is significantly progressively productive if you extravagant it.)

7. Outdoor bicycling: Approximately 680 calories for each hour biking at a fast, lively pace will raise your pulse, regardless of whether you are outside or inside. Add to some rocky landscape and mountains and gets significantly more calorie consuming.

The volume of calories devoured is straightforwardly proportionate to the measure of sustenance, just like the kind of nourishment an individual expends. The best way to lessen calories is by being cautious about what you devour and captivating in dynamic physical exercises to consume overabundance calories in your body.

A Guide to Mindful Eating

Keeping up a contemporary, quick-paced way of life can leave a brief period to oblige your necessities. You are moving always starting with one thing then onto the next, not focusing on what your psyche or body truly needs. Rehearsing mindfulness can help you to comprehend those necessities.

When eating mindfulness is connected, it can help you recognize your examples and practices while simultaneously standing out to appetite and completion related to body signs.

Originating from the act of pressure decrease dependent on mindfulness, rehearsing mindfulness while eating can help you focus on the present minute instead of proceeding with ongoing and unacceptable propensities.

Careful eating is an approach to begin an internal looking course to help you become increasingly aware of your nourishment association and utilize that information to eat with joy.

The body conveys a great deal of information and information, so you can start settling on cognizant choices as opposed to falling into programmed — and regularly feeling driven — practices when you apply attention to the eating knowledge.

You are better prepared to change your conduct once you become aware of these propensities.

Individuals that need to be cautious about sustenance and nourishment are asked to:

- Explore their inward knowledge about sustenance— different preferences

- Choose sustenance that please and support their bodies

- Accept explicit sustenance inclinations without judgment or self-analysis

- Practice familiarity with the indications of their bodies beginning to eat and quit eating.

General Principles of Mindful Eating

One methodology to careful eating depends on the core values given by Rebecca J. Frey, Ph.D., and Laura Jean Cataldo, RN: tune in to the internal craving and satiety signs of your body Identify private triggers for careless eating, for example, social weights, amazing sentiments, and explicit nourishments.

Here are a couple of tips for getting you started.

- Start with one meal. It requires some investment to begin with any new propensity. It very well may be difficult to make cautious eating rehearses constantly. However, you can practice with one dinner or even a segment of a supper. Attempt to focus on appetite sign and sustenance choices before you start eating or sinking into the feelings of satiety toward the part of the arrangement—these are phenomenal approaches to begin a routine with regards to consideration.

- Remove view distractions place or turn off your phone in another space. Mood killers such the TV and PC and set away whatever else —, for example, books, magazines, and papers—that can divert you from eating. Give the feast before your complete consideration.

- Tune in your perspective when you start this activity, become aware of your attitude. Perceive that there is no right or off base method for eating, yet simply unmistakable degrees of eating background awareness. Focus your consideration on eating sensations. When you understand that your brain has meandered, take it delicately back to the eating knowledge.

- Draw in your senses with this activity. There are numerous approaches to explore. Attempt to investigate one nourishment thing utilizing every one of your faculties. When you put sustenance in your mouth, see the scents, surfaces, hues, and flavors. Attempt to see how the sustenance changes as you cautiously bite each nibble.

- Take as much time as necessary. Eating cautiously includes backing off, enabling your stomach related hormones to tell your mind that you are finished before eating excessively. It's a fabulous method to hinder your fork between chomps. Additionally, you will be better arranged to value your supper experience, especially in case you're with friends and family.

Rehearsing mindfulness in a bustling globe can be trying now and again; however, by knowing and applying these essential core values and techniques, you can discover approaches to settle your body all the more promptly. When you figure out how much your association with nourishment can adjust to improve things, you will be charmingly astounded — and this can importantly affect your general prosperity and wellbeing.

Formal dinners, be that as it may, will, in general, assume a lower priority about occupied ways of life for generally people. Rather, supper times are an opportunity to endeavor to do each million stuff in turn. Consider having meals at your work area or accepting your Instagram fix over breakfast to control through a task.

The issue with this is you are bound to be genuinely determined in your decisions about healthy eating and eat excessively on the off chance that you don't focus on the nourishment you devour or the way you eat it.

That is the place mindfulness goes in. You can apply similar plans to a yoga practice straight on your lunch plate". Cautious eating can enable you to tune in to the body's information of what, when, why, and the amount to eat," says Lynn Rossy, Ph.D., essayist of The Mindfulness-Based Eating Solution and the Center for Mindful Eating director. "Rather than relying upon another person (or an eating routine) to reveal to you how to eat, developing a minding association with your own body can achieve tremendous learning and change."

From the ranch to the fork — can help you conquer enthusiastic eating, make better nourishment choices, and even experience your suppers in a crisp and ideally better way. To make your next dinner mindful, pursue these measures.

The Mindful Eating Diet

Being obvious, eating reliably alone isn't an eating regimen. No extreme purifying, no expulsion of specific fixings, no clearing of pantries, no prevailing fashions, and no quick fixes. Cautious eating can be utilized as a system to help manage increasingly cautious nourishment choices that could prompt weight reduction, even though it is important that at whatever point we pick sustenance dependent on a specific outcome, we don't eat mindfully — we eat with an unfortunate obligation that is perhaps reckless.

Essentially careful eating urges us to be available while cooking or eating, empowering us to enjoy our sustenance with no judgment truly, blame, uneasiness, or inside a remark. Regular eating routine culture makes a lot of our eating pressure, carrying with it a pile of weight, power, and false desires. Accordingly, a large number of us will, in general, consider nourishment to be a reward or

punishment.

Chapter 9 How To Boost Your Motivation To Work Out

There are two major components of weight loss; your diet and your daily activities. To lose weight, you should eat just enough food to keep you energized for your daily activities.

In this chapter, we will focus on building your motivation to keep exercising. Keeping an active lifestyle will increase your metabolic rate. It will make your body burn more energy even when you are resting.

To be able to integrate workouts to your lifestyle however, you should make sure that you enjoy them. If it feels too much like work, it will be too difficult to maintain. There will come a time that your mind will be defeated by the distractions and temptations around you.

How To Build Motivation For Working Out:

Set Realistic Goals And Make A Plan To Reach Them

Before you can start lifting weights, jogging or doing other types of activities, you should put in writing what you want to achieve. If you want to lose weight, you should set the exact number of pounds that you want to lose and the amount of time that you have to achieve your goal. You could also set your goals on specific body parts like your waistline or your arms.

Following the S.M.A.R.T. philosophy to set goals is an ideal tool to use. This ensures goals are Specific, Measurable, Attainable, Realistic and have a Timeline. You should then find a workout plan that fits your schedule and your personality. You should consider the time that you have for your workouts and the effort that you can devote to it.

Remind Yourself Of The Benefits Of Working Out

Being aware of the benefits of working out will help you continue to do it. You will also be able to build your will power to avoid being lazy. This will remind you that you are not doing this just to look great but also to become healthier.

Make A List Of Activities That You Enjoy

If you love dancing, you should include that into your workout plan. If you prefer sports, you should train for the type of sport that you want to participate in. By doing things that you like, you will be able to transition to an active lifestyle with much more ease.

Include A Variety Of Activities In Your Workout Plan

Aside from doing what you love, you should also make it habit to try new things and to vary the activities in your workout plan. Lifting weights or running all the time will become boring after some time. If your body is not presented with a challenge every time, it will no longer improve.

Prepare The Necessary Equipment And Outfits

Spending for your workout plan is like investing in your body; you will be expecting a return on your investment. Not only will you feel like an athlete, but this will make you work harder and become more disciplined in following your strategies.

Make Your Workouts A Social Activity

You should avoid doing everything by yourself. Just like in your diet plan, you should also include the people around you. Join people who also like to work out. Motivation, enthusiasm and positive thinking are contagious. You will have a better chance of continuing your weight loss program if you have these people around.

Analyze The Factors That Motivate You

You should also use your metacognitive abilities to improve your performance. Every time you feel extra motivated, you should analyze the internal and external sources of your motivation. Being aware of these factors will give you insights about how your mind works. You can use some of these factors to stimulate your motivation when you are feeling down.

Reward Yourself For Reaching Your Goals

Rewards are things that you allow yourself to have when you reach a certain goal. They are expected to increase the likelihood that you will repeat your positive behaviors. You should decide on the rewards that you will give yourself when making your goals. The thought of the reward will help motivate you. In times when the workout routine becomes hard, you should remind yourself of the reward that you will get if you push through.

You should make sure however, you will be able to follow through with your promise. The most important promises are the ones that you give to yourself.

Recharge Your Motivation to Exercise

The only thing that is standing between you and the body you want is mental blocks so, to get over those speed bumps and avoid the inevitable excuses, follow these top methods for rebooting your workout and your mental and emotional state.

You Think – my scales are stuck, why am I bothering?

Rethink - This podge will go

Stick with it. Weight loss is never consistent and the scales, unless they are cheap or faulty, will never lie. First off, the more weight you have to lose, the quicker it will come off – IN THE BEGINNING. After that, it will all start to slow down. Most people reach a weight loss plateau, where they don't lose any weight for several weeks and it is at this point that you must not give in.

One more important point – do not weight yourself every day, it's a very bad habit. Your weight will go up and down daily but it will go down overall. Weigh yourself once a week or fortnight.

That way, any loss in weight is a much bigger motivator. Weighing yourself daily is the best way to demotivate yourself so don't do it. Just because you aren't losing any pounds, doesn't mean that your body isn't losing inches and the only way to tell that is how your clothes fit. Give yourself plenty of credit for how much better you look and use that as your motivation to continue.

Redo - Move your routine up a gear

As you lose weight, your metabolism will alter to accommodate the lighter smaller you. That means you are going to have to change the way you encourage your body to burn fat and shed pounds. If you are already on a light diet of around 1500 calories a day, don't cut any more off. Instead, make your workouts more intense and work out for a bit longer each time. Not only will this result in more calories being burned off, it will also make your cardio capacity much larger. This means that you will find it easier to exercise and will be motivated to work out for just that little bit longer. Crank up the resistance on the stationery bike, set the treadmill at more of an incline, walk for a bit longer than you do now, walk at a faster pace or go for one-minute interval runs. Between toning exercises, fit in a set of jumping jacks, running on the spot or step-ups.

You Think - I really can't manage another rep

Rethink - Don't my biceps look fantastic!

If you need a motivational boost, a bit of a lift, psych yourself up mentally and emotionally while you are training. This can increase your muscle power by up to 8% s well as their size and bigger muscles result in an increase in metabolism, which burns off fat faster. So if you needed just one bit of motivation, there it is. Mental imagery is a wonderful boost – when your arms or legs feel tired, imagine bigger and stronger muscles, tell yourself how great you look and you will get another rep or two out.

Redo – Take it down a notch

If you really can manage another rep at the same rate, lighten things off a bit. If you are lifting weights, knock the weights down by 10% until you know you can do another rep in good form. If you are sprinting circuits, slow it down for the last one. The more effort you put in, the better the rewards will be so, even if your final rep is at a lower rate than the previous ones, it's still more effort and it will reap rewards. Don't ever beat yourself up if you can't do it but keep this in mind – pushing your limits a little further will get you results you never dreamed of seeing.

You Think - I can't run a mile!

Rethink – That jogger looks like Brad Pitt/Angelina Jolie – whoever takes your fancy at the time really!

When you are slogging your way through that mile, turn your thinking to what is going on around you. Yes, you may slow down a little but you will keep on going and you will finish that mile. Repeat a mental mantra over and over again – something like "I am a running machine" and you will find that you can go for longer and further.

Redo – Divide and Conquer

If you are running a mile, to start with split it up into some bits running and some walking. Jog for maybe quarter of a mile and the walk for a further half mile before jogging the final stretch. As you get better and fitter, as well as leaner, you can jog for further and gradually cut down the walking time. If you can do this three times a week, it won't take long before you can run the entire mile. Your motivation? Your fitness and how you look. Think about how much better you feel and you will keep on going. Do set up a routine for running though. If you only go as and when, it will not work.

You Think - I've damaged my knee/leg/arm etc., I won't be able to do any exercise for a month

Rethink – Where did I put that Pilates DVD?

If you injure yourself and stop working out, it takes a maximum of three days for your body to start losing its conditioning. If that isn't enough motivation of you to get up and go, tell yourself this – there's more than one way to reach that goal. Start by making a list of all the negative thoughts you are having and then turn them into positive thoughts. For example, "I can't go to my exercise class tonight, everything I've done will all go to waste" could be turned into "oh well, now I can start using that Pilates DVD I bought".

Redo – Switch things out

Your regular exercise class might be out but there are other options that are low or no impact. Depending on what injury you have sustained, a bit of moderate training on the elliptical bike can burn off up to 416 calories a hour, water jogging can bur 512 calories an hour as can cycling. These are all good alternatives but only if your injury allows it. If you can't exercise because your legs are injured or you have knee pain, you can still exercise the upper part of your body with hand weights. You can still sit on a chair and punch a boxing bag and Pilates is a form of exercise that is gentle yet effective, designed to allow the maximum benefits in a safe way.

You Think – Spinning classes are way too intense for my liking

Rethink – That guy over there in the Lycra shorts doesn't look as tough as he thinks

We are afraid of the unknown, of what we don't know so before you dismiss a particular exercise out of hand, have a go. You might just find that you enjoy it. Watch a class first, right from the start. If you see a spinning class from the middle onwards, the pace and the sweat are going to put you off but if you see it from the beginning, you might just find that it not that bad.

Redo - Find your own pace

With most exercise classes, you are in control of how it makes you feel. Just because the rest of the class is throwing themselves about or the other runners on the track are sprinting all the way does not mean that you have to. If there comes a point in the class where the instructor tells you to increase resistance, only go as far as you are comfortable going. If you get tired and can't keep up, slow things down a bit. The idea of exercise is to get the hang of doing it correctly and safely and to have fun. Go into each class telling yourself that you are there to enjoy yourself and you will.

You Think - I can only exercise at home, that's not going to work!

Rethink - There really is no place like home!

The first thing you have do is work out what tis going to motivate you to get off the couch and stay off. Then you need to come up with a plan that is going to put you in the frame of mind to commit to exercising at home. Get your workout clothes on when you get home from work or first thing in the morning so that you know you are going to exercise and you get into the right mindset. Create a schedule that has accountability in it. For example, get a friend to come round on certain days and do those kickboxing or fitness DVD's.

Redo – Get a takeaway

And I don't mean a fast food one. If you can't afford to join a gym, you can have one beamed into you lounge for a fraction of the cost. Using email and website, personal trainers are there to help you without you having to leave your own home. Some of them will provide you with a customized routine to follow as well as a diet plan.

You Think - I can't stay on that cardio machine for more than 30 minutes, it's like a form of slow torture!

Rethink - Who's going to be sent home tonight on BB/Jungle/X-Factor, etc.

When you are on the treadmill don't waste time thinking about the exercise you are doing, it won't work. Instead, turn to other things, like watching your favorite TV program, or plug into your music and lose yourself. You might just be surprised at how fast the time goes and how much more you achieve when your mind is elsewhere.

Redo – Work first, rest later

Plan your routine so that you start hard, fast, and slow down towards the end. If you start off with high intensity workouts and then go on down to lower intensity, especially on the treadmill, you will find that more fat is burned and your workout won't feel quite so stressful. Your motivation is that you know you can finish light and not absolutely worn out, dripping sweat, feeling like you couldn't move another step if you wanted to. Try this 45-minute plan – warm up for 5 minutes at a nice easy pace. Increase speed up to a moderate level and for 20 minutes increase your speed or incline by 1% for every 2 minutes. Then lower the incline and/or the speed slightly for 15 minutes followed by five minute at a nice easy cool-down pace.

You Think – I haven't go the energy after work to exercise

Rethink - just 10 minutes, that's all

There is a huge difference between mental and physical tiredness and. Believe it or not, physical activity can knock mental fatigue into touch. Tell yourself that you will do just 10 minutes and you will find, more often than not, that you end up doing more, simply because once you get going, your tiredness and fatigue disappears. Not only that, your mood improves too.

Redo – Stack it in your favor

When you leave work to go home, make sure your route goes past your gym. The sight of people exercising is often motivation enough so make sure you have your workout gear with you. Not only that, you can give yourself a big pat on the back for having taken time out to exercise, instead of going home and flopping on the sofa. If you don't feel like a full gym workout, have an alternative plan in place. Get off the train or the bus a stop earlier or have your workout mat already set up in front of the TV and the workout DVD ready to go. If you have an alternative plan in place, you are twice as likely to have the motivation to work out and you are twice as likely to actually do something instead of opting for the easy get-out.

It is very easy for me to tell you to learn to see things in a more positive light but that is exactly what you have to do. When something negative pops into your mind, change it for a positive thought. Think of another way of doing something. If you really cant get to the gym, exercise at home instead of giving it a miss altogether. Tell yourself that you can do those extra few minutes, that you can push yourself that little bit further.

Conclusion

You look in the mirror and you are dissatisfied. Do you wish that your shape, your nose, your legs, your hair were like somebody else's? Why do we always compare ourselves? Why aren't we reconciled with our appearance? We have heard ad nauseam that we should love ourselves, despite our mistakes or flaws. This includes things related to our personality as well as our bodies. However, there are very few people who can accept and be content with themselves. It is not about not wanting to change. It is a commendable endeavor when one wants to achieve or retain their looks or care about looking more attractive.

At the same time, most people are much more critical, more strict with themselves than justified. They are continuously dissatisfied with themselves and don't see in the mirror what others see. Some girls feel a significant discomfort looking at each other, both because they don't like looking at each other in general, and because they don't like what they see. Where do these reactions come from?

What usually happens is that you don't look at yourself; you only see yourself with respect to that ideal of beauty that you have in your head. This is where dissatisfaction creeps in. It has to do with the theory of social confrontation. We compare ourselves with those we consider better than ourselves; self-esteem is negatively affected. We all have a model in the head, a term of comparison that we have built by looking at years of magazines, advertising, and movies with perfect Hollywood princesses. The mantra must become one and only one: there is no need for me to compare myself to that model because everybody is a unique, generous specimen, rich in the indications of what I am.

Life would be much simpler and happier if we could accept ourselves as we are. A lot of negative emotions would be released, we would have less stress, and more of the things that really matter come into view. The bottom line is, if we really need to change something, we can't do it until we make peace with the current state. This is a vicious circle.

The mind works, in effect, in a strange way. If we resist something, we get more of it.

After all, if we focus our attention on what is bad, we reinforce the bad. And what we pay the most attention to as we think about something will come true.

Everything that comes from you that relates to you is just yours: your feelings, your voice, your actions, your ears, your thighs, your hopes and fears. That's why you are unique. Be happy that you are different from anyone, that you look the way you do and that it is just you. Start to feel that it's your own body, not something separate that you need to live with.

Do you want your house to be just like anyone else's? Or do you love the little things that carry memories? Don't you love the atmosphere of your messy place after playing with your kids? And the plain curtain that you know you should replace, but which your mom sewed and looks so good? Or the piece of furniture that everyone says you should throw out, but you insist on it?

That's how you should feel about your body. You should understand that you don't need to compare it with anyone else's because it's impossible to compare unique things. In addition, who determines what beautiful and ugly mean? You should not compare your body to the celebrities' perfect-looking bodies. First, because they are adjusted with Photoshop and other programs, and they are not real. Second, because you are different, as is everybody.

You're not them. You are neither the next-door girl who, after three children, looks like she did at twenty, nor your friend who you think is gorgeous. You should not only accept your body, but you should fall in love with it. Do you think like Bonnie? Do you think no one could love you because you have some extra weight? Then ask yourself the following questions. Could you fall in love with someone only if they are perfect looking? Would you really love someone because of their body? I'll go further.

Do we really love perfect looking people? I bet you prefer your imperfect companion instead of a perfect looking bodybuilder. You like the little faults of your wife, husband, kids, and friends because they belong to you too. We love imperfections better than perfections.

See? We don't measure people based on their weight. In addition, if you are happy with your body and your existence, it will also manifest in your radiance.

How should you love your body?

Sandra Díaz Ferrer, a researcher at the University of Granada, works with women who do not like their bodies and suffer from eating disorders. After years of observations, she published a study in the Journal of Behavior Therapy and Experimental Psychiatry, which reveals how looking at the mirror correctly can help in the treatment of bulimia nervosa. Her technique can be fundamental for all women dissatisfied with their image, or those who suffer from eating disorders. Imagine you have a fear of bugs that obsesses you. The psychologist might ask you to look closely at bugs until you get used to them, desensitizing yourself to the features that first terrified you. You can apply the same procedure to your body (Ferrer, 2015).

Here's an exercise that can help those who struggle to be happy about their own imperfections. You have to stand in front of a large mirror and look at yourself as if you were doing it for the first time in your life, like never before, taking time for yourself. It must be a constructive and very careful observation. No distractions, no work commitments, no notification to pull your attention. Only you and the mirror. Next time you hate your body or any part of your body, stand in front of a mirror and look at yourself. Go from top to bottom and sort out your "mistakes". You will have to start looking at yourself from head to toe, objectively observing all the details, without comparisons or judgments.

- Remember what that part of your body has done for you. When did it help, when did it protect you, when did it do something physically useful for you? Say thank you for something that was of help to you. Learn to practice gratitude.

- Appreciate what you have and love your inner self. Don't let a scale or a size define your identity and skills. It is no use to criticize yourself fiercely when looking in the mirror.

Here are some ways to cultivate enormous gratitude in everyday life. When faced with a negative situation, do not be discouraged. Ask yourself instead what you can learn for the future and for reasons to feel grateful. Promise yourself not to be negative or not to criticize yourself for three days. If you make a mistake, forgive yourself and go on your way. This exercise will help you understand that negative thoughts are just a waste of energy. Every day, list the reasons why you feel grateful. The body is a miracle and you should celebrate all the gifts it has given you. Think about the goals you have passed, your relationships and the activities you love: it was your body that allowed you to do all this. Take note of it every day. Go to the next body part and do the same.

When you have reached your toes, return to your head again, to your face, and now, going downhill, just say to all your body parts, "I love you." Even if you feel a little stupid about it, don't stop. You see, you're going to have a completely different relationship with your appearance. And by the way, let's not forget, it's not a coincidence that it's called outer. What's inside is more important. But what's inside is visible outside. So use your inner self to love your outer, and you will be much calmer, happier, more satisfied and more confident.

Set the alarm and watch yourself for at least 40 minutes at a time. Doing so could change your life. Experts talk about the epidemic spread of body image disorder, a severe problem that leads us to see ourselves as inadequate every time we look at our body. According to research, 90.2% of women have an altered image of themselves and are not satisfied with their bodies, a fact that has a lot to do with how we look in the mirror. The mirror is your new weapon: from enemy to ally, but learning to use it in the right way (Ferrer, 2015).

Compliment yourself. You should consider yourself and treat yourself with the same kindness and the same admiration that you would reserve for those you love. You probably wouldn't direct the same criticisms you do to yourself, to another person. Don't hesitate to compliment yourself, don't be too hard on yourself and forgive yourself when you make a mistake. Get rid of the hatred you feel for yourself, replace it with greater understanding and appreciation. Look in the mirror and repeat: "I am attractive. I am sure of myself. I am fantastic!" Do it regularly and you'll begin to see yourself in a positive light. When you reach a goal, be proud. Look in the mirror and say, "Great job, I'm proud of myself."

Stay away from negativity. Avoid people who only talk badly about their bodies. You risk getting infected by their insecurities and dwelling on your faults. Life is too short and valuable to be consumed by hating yourself or looking for every little fault, especially when the perception you have of yourself tends to be much more critical than that of others. If a person starts to criticize their body, don't get involved in their negativity. Change the subject instead or leave. Wear comfortable clothes that reflect who you are. Everything you have in the wardrobe should enhance your body. Don't wear uncomfortable clothes just to impress others. Remember that those who accept themselves always look great. Wear clean, undamaged garments to dress the body the way you deserve. Buy matching briefs and bras, even though you are the only one to see them. You will remind your inner self that you are doing it exclusively for yourself.

Ask others what they love about you and what they consider your best qualities. This will help you develop yourself and remind you that your body has given you so much. You will probably be surprised to discover what others find beautiful about you, you have probably forgotten about them.

Surround yourself with people who love themselves. People absorb the attitudes and behaviors of the people around them. If your life is full of positive influences, you will also adopt them, and they will help you to love both your inner and outer. Look for optimistic people who work hard to achieve their goals and respect themselves.

Think of all the people who have reached important goals and whom you admire. They can be individuals you know personally or not. They are probably renowned and respected for the goals achieved regardless of the type of physique they have. Take the opportunity to remember that the body is not an obstacle to living or finding happiness. The body can help you pursue all your dreams and desires.

Think of your family, your closest friends, or a person you don't know personally but have always admired. Make a list of their best qualities. Then ask yourself if the image they have of themselves or their bodies has positively influenced their successes or prevented them from reaching a goal.